CONTENTS

My BeaST MODE playlist, in no particular order.

This book is dedicated to my family and friends, first and foremost. They have my back, just as I have theirs and I know that will never change.

I, I'm a new day rising

I'm a brand new sky

to hang the stars upon tonight.

-TIMES LIKE THESE, DAVE GROHL,
THE FOO FIGHTERS

MIDDLE CLASS CANCER AND OTHER NATURAL DISASTERS

A LOVE LETTER

By Dr. Shannon M. Mulvey

INTRODUCTION

This is the story of one woman's journey -- a woman who walked out of work on a summer Friday afternoon to go to a routine mammogram, a medical appointment which she assumed would be like any other, just something to cross off her list of busy things to do, so she could get back to taking care of the trivial business of being a working mother. "Not trivial," you say? It is to her now. Oh, the working part is not trivial, the mothering part is not trivial. But take both of those things away and what is left?

Imagine an appointment that changed the course of her life so greatly that immediately going back to work was not an option. That she would see her kids with expressions on their faces that she had never seen on them before, expressions of despair and fear. Imagine standing before her world as it crumbled and pretending to be strong, because her kids had to know she would not back down from the unexpected crisis. She doesn't know how she got through that moment of telling them for the first time. There will forever be a line in their family's sand, the "before the breast cancer diagnosis" and the "after breast cancer diagnosis."

This is the story of a bad dream, the one that makes you wake up gasping for breath and you take a few moments to realize -- oh, thank God, it was only a dream. And you settle yourself back to sleep a little cozier and a little more thankful for what you have.

Except this time it wasn't a bad dream. It was reality and it needed to be faced. There was no choice. Stand when you are weak, get control of your heart beating out of your chest. Tell your kids, "Your life will not change. I will not change. I will still be the same mom telling you to pick up your dirty socks. You will still get to your swim practices, your Little League games, but it might not be the way it has always been for a little while."

Change is good they say. No, she disagrees. This change was not good. At least not initially and not for a long time afterward.

She had spent nearly twenty years as a holistic practitioner. She had spent thirteen years as a natural childbirth instructor. She was used to teaching, hoping that her clients left her with a little golden nugget of knowledge that they didn't have before. That daily goal was now an immediate loss. She had to be taken care of now. The impatience, the frustration, showed and she knew it did. Something had been stolen from her, which could not be given back.

She heard a lot of people say, "They say God doesn't give you what you can't handle," but she knew in her heart she wasn't handling it with the grace and sophistication she would have liked. But how could she when she was on the floor? Another phrase that people take out of their pocket in times of distress -- "that which does not kill you makes you stronger." A person on their knees has no idea how to reply to this platitude. They don't feel strong; they didn't ever ask to prove their strength. Another gem -- "everything happens for a reason." People have no idea what to say and she can appreciate their attempts to make her feel better. Nobody ever promised her a rose garden.

And, almost two years later, she can almost see a glimmer of why this may have happened for a reason, but she doesn't accept it as a happy accident. She almost doesn't accept it at all. It reeks of unfairness. And she tried to look for the silver linings. She really did. About nine months after her diagnosis, she excitedly accepted an invitation to a morning question and answer session with "Mom Bosses," hoping to hear the secrets of these successful working moms.

She waited patiently to ask the question spinning in her head while they imparted their secrets. These mom-bosses certainly had a vision of what they wanted to do with their lives. In her brain, she kind of realized that they had the cushion of money behind them. They were married to professional athletes, financial gurus or practitioners in specialized fields of medicine.

Their drive simply came from what would feel good to them to be successful in their hobbies or their passions.

The question and answer session wrapped up before she could ask her question. There was a "thank you for coming, we hope you all enjoyed the women on our panel and their tips for being your own mom boss." Or something like that. But her hand had still been raised. She ended up blurting out her question. "But, wait!! What if you had a dream and you were living it and you got so blown off course that you couldn't see it through?" She HAD been a Mom Boss, she could have given a class on making it work in her prior life that she was still mourning.

She didn't know that all along, her daily routine had been fragile like a revered piece of antique china. She counted her blessings every night, surely. But, in one moment in time, she now had the shards of her life in her hands and on the floor and on the walls. The break was explosive, complete. And whenever something fragile breaks, you know that there will be pieces you can't find, that skitter away, preventing you from being able to glue it back together. A lady behind her murmured, "I'm so glad you asked that question." The panel looked at her and said, "Well, you just have to find your passion."

But, how? When she had HAD a passion? "Make a dream board!" one panelist said. Ummmm, her life had fallen apart. She was trying to find the pieces. There was not enough glue in the entire world to glue Humpty-Dumpty back together again. Except now she was supposed to sit and cut images out of magazines that she hoped to attain someday. Didn't the mom bosses understand? She had no time for cutting and pasting. She was trying to feed the kids, see to their needs, stop the foreclosure on her home due to medical bills, explore bankruptcy, while losing her entire salary towards their previously dual income (by necessity) household. There was no time for arts and crafts. She and her family were poised to lose everything they had worked so hard to achieve.

This is my story, unaffectionately referred to as, "Middle Class Cancer and Other Natural Disasters. A Love Story." Because, indeed, there was love. Big, huge puddles of ostentatious love. People caught her when she fell, and I did fall. You had already figured out it was me, right? I am that woman.

Oh, don't get me wrong, I DID make a dreamboard. I was hoping it would help. And, I think maybe it did. But middle class cancer patients don't have nannies and cleaning ladies and landscapers. While I fought for my life and our family fought to keep any semblance of their former realities, there was food to be bought and made, there was a house to be cleaned and a yard to maintain. There were bills to be paid and tests to be signed and carpools to keep up. There were calls, tons and tons of calls, often sitting on hold, hoping that the person on the other end of the line could see how unhelpful they were.

Strangely enough, a favorite gift to give a cancer patient is an adult coloring book. Oh, my God, I'm so sorry -- you thought I would have time to color? You thought that coloring might relieve the massive burden of stress she has found herself under? I'm sorry. I have no time to color. I'm trying to save my family and my house and the life that we knew, complete with a $10,000 deductible and a $20,000 out of network deductible.

This story is my journey, often dictated into my phone from a chemotherapy chair, trying desperately to forget that poison was being dripped into my arm. Or it was dictated from the radiation table, to keep me from crying, because tears that fall when I lay on my back annoy my face. I threw myself into trying to teach someone something. Any someone, any something. Like I used to do at work, like is part of my identity, just as I was born with brown hair and green eyes. I love to teach.

These chapters were written in real time. They are raw, I can sometimes barely go back and read them: it's equivalent to going back to read your diary, years later, except to see words that, viscerally, can put me back right there again, scared for my life. It can bring me back to my husband and I lying in our bed, in the dark of night, when the house was quiet, both staring at the ceiling, holding hands, afraid to say what was going through our minds, the "what if 'until death do us part' is soon?" And he always knew when I had started crying and embraced me.

It is my hope that the woman sitting in the chemo chair, facing the future loss of her breast on a known date coming on the calendar, will feel understood. It is my hope that her best friend will realize just what she needs from my words. My best friend Googled "How to be a best friend to your best friend with a new, scary diagnosis" and she later said to me, when I thanked her for understanding that I couldn't always get back to her, using her charming southern drawl, "Girl?" (An aside, the word "girl," in a southern drawl sometimes may take several minutes to finish uttering) "Girrrrrrrllllllll? I actually looked up what I should do and one of the things said to not expect a call back. But that I should call you anyway, to tell you that I love you and I'm think-ing of you, so that's what I did."

Another best friend worried, "Oh!! I feel so bad! I didn't Goo-gle anything like that!" Don't feel bad, my friend -- you sent a package to me every day for three weeks, in order for me to feel your love. Still other best friends appointed themselves the captains of my team. Team Shannon was born from their gen-erosity of time and spirit and they immediately went to work selling Team Shannon t-shirts and bracelets to help stave off the financial strain that we were facing. And there were gifts of food and love and casseroles and gas station gift cards.

It is also my hope that you can know exactly what your loved one is going through and what she may need, or as close as you possibly can. The truth in advertising is that she is completely deranged. Like a feral, wild animal that has now been caged; you will understand that she only feels horror and fear, but someday she'll be back. Please be patient with her. That's what she needs. It is my hope that someone interested in the human experience will be entertained, enlightened. And, finally, it is my hope that somebody, somewhere learns something that they didn't know before. That's all I have ever wanted.

It's hard to put that on a dream board, but I'll be on the lookout for an image that might possibly represent that drive of mine to teach. Let me know if you see something that I could use.

* * *

DIAGNOSIS

<u>Just Waiting on a Train...</u>

What a year -- 2017 will certainly be remembered as a standout year here -- I had turned 45. I had my first cup of coffee, ever. The coffee shop thought I said coffee, and not " hot tea.' Those who know me know I only like tea. I got my first pair of reading glasses and I have a new level of empathy for those of you who have struggled with poor eyesight your whole lives. While I didn't feel "done" raising my kids, far from it, they had become a lot more (sometimes just a little bit more) independent. With my youngest now turning eight, I felt like I had achieved more of an even keel. So I started making plans, like maybe I could find time to read more than two books in a year again? Or could I maybe make a trip to swim in blue waters again?

I was a latecomer to Facebook and I had complained for a long time about why I would NEVER want to be on there. I said things like, "You were never supposed to have all of your friends for your whole life." Or, "If they want to reach out to me, they can call me." Or, more indignantly, "This was originally about boys critiquing girls' looks." I think I picked that nugget up from Gwyneth Paltrow at some point.

But I got curious about my friends, I missed you guys!! And you were there!! I've been running like HELL over these years and

I've lost touch with alot of you -- my most fun finding was hearing my sorority sisters' senses of humor through their Facebook banter. It was almost like living in the house again! I didn't have to look for you, you found me! Each one of your personalities has shown through. I have tons of incriminating pictures that

I thought I could start artfully placing... 😄 I got excited about perhaps going to our 25 year reunion, to KJ's September party... and I loved having instant access to my Cub Scout troop and my Girl Scout troop through our secret Facebook pages. It turns out you younger moms didn't really answer my emails, but you responded on Facebook instantly! It was instant gratification!

I now KNEW I could expect my scouts on the field trips I planned for our troops, so I let myself get a little inspired, plan some more fun into my days. Everybody who knows me knows I love working. I love what I do; but I realized I was missing out on some really fun things.

So I started making plans! I was able to work some more flexibility into my work hours. I've been teaching natural childbirth and breastfeeding classes for about 13 years, and as much as I had a passion to teach these (I have LOVED it like crazy), I realized that my family needed me more, so I started making space. I regretfully gave up teaching, but I knew it was the right time and I felt blessed to have taught over 350 couples in those 13 years. The thought of all of your babies out there, with parents making healthy choices for them, ALWAYS makes me so, so happy.

But 2017 brought me something else instead; changed all of these plans instantly... I didn't know what I had been making "space" for, and now I do.

An emergency mammogram in the beginning of the month (I no longer like the alliteration of what 7/7/17 sounds like) brought a doctor into the room who related that I had a mass on my breast, multiple, in fact. It was a Friday night, 5 PM...

I was shocked. I brought no one with me because I wasn't expecting any bad news. I was scheduled for four biopsies within 2-1/2 days of that appointment, which confirmed an ugly diagnosis... metastatic invasive ductal carcinoma.

It is considered "inflammatory".

My two older sons were leaving for Boy Scout camp that week.

We didn't want to lay it on them before they left -- we didn't want them to have to deal with this information by themselves. We wanted to give this information to all of our children together, in both a developmentally appropriate way, but also in the comfort of their home, so they had the freedom to process it as they needed.

So I cried that week, waiting for them to come home. I cried behind doors and in bathrooms. I told my little ones that I was getting a head cold, I told them I had mascara in my eyes, I told them I had just heard an emotional song. Anything to get through that first week. We told them all the following Saturday. All the medical interventions in the world didn't compare to having to sit down and tell them this news.

My first response to my diagnosis was disbelief. I have no family history; I have no risk factors. I've now been tested for the gene, which I do not have. I've been eating organically for over 15 years, I run a veggie co-op! I BUY alkaline water on purpose! I am a holistic practitioner, I do yoga, I get 10,000 steps, I got rid of my microwave ten years ago, I make green smoothies! I breast-fed four babies, a known cancer fighter, for four years, plus one and a half months.

This was my first way of attacking this cancer, by making the list of why it's impossible for me to have! It's a really, really, really long list. I'll spare you the details. And yet I do have it, so I turn to this list to help me realize that I am not a number, I am not a statistic and hopefully these reasons of why it's "impossible" for me to get cancer will be the reasons why I beat cancer. I didn't live in fear of cancer, but given the choice between A and B, I always chose the A. I started spewing in my head -- this is so incredibly impossible, that maybe it really is! And I will wake up from this bad dream. Anger was my most prominent emotion in the first three weeks following diagnosis.

We are not being quiet about this. It is not a secret. And, in some ways, I thought I could now use Facebook a lot differently than I had originally thought. Because I am interested in hearing from people who have navigated these rough waters. I'm not going to lie, it took two weeks to peel myself off the floor. It took two weeks to be able to go out in public and not break down if somebody said a kind word, which I have greatly appreciated, but I couldn't guarantee a polite, controlled response.

Dr. Shannon M. Mulvey

Many of the people I talk to tell me that cancer doesn't kill people -- that depression does. These people don't know my usual love of life... I really do laugh my head off all the time! I see the humor in life! There are many people that say to cry, get it out. And that has not been my business plan, either -- it has just been impossible not to.

I have learned that my tumor markers are considered "triple positive." The medical feedback I have gotten seems to indicate that I am "lucky" because of this designation, as long as it is no where else in my body. We hope to have a definitive answer of that this week, but we are hopeful.

We immediately reached out to our kids' friends' parents, I had an email prepared that I sent out the moment we told our kids. We knew that we were going to need help and the response has been amazing.

First, by my husband, Tom, and my family. They don't let me go to an appointment alone. My mother, and my sister have dropped everything to make that happen.

Last night, our neighbors/friends got our kids in on a secret and they all appeared at our house wearing "Team Shannon" bracelets. They walked up with their hands behind their backs and there was a brief second that I thought I was about to get hit by water balloons or pies in the face.

Instead they presented their wrists with pink "Team Shannon" bracelets on, with an icon of a lighthouse. Our kids got us into a crazy hobby. We've gone to the top of 74 lighthouses at this point. I now consider them all beacons of hope! But I can't believe I have a team! Me! You all know my level of commitment to sports! 😂

A friend in my veggie co-op asked if she could run in my honor in the Avon 39 mile walk in October. That offer brought me to my knees.

I came home to a dozen pink roses one night, from another friend saying that I've "got this."

The people I fell on immediately heard me having a hysterical reaction to not having any ponytail holders. I am now the owner of hundreds. It's your regular list of things to do, when you thought you'd be able to stop and get to them sometime this week - these little tiny things that people took care were actually enormous gifts in my eyes.

My place of employment, they have never put any pressure on me and have only offered up love, prayers and support. I even hate to say "place of employment." We think of ourselves as a family there. I walked out of work that day to go to my appointment and I told my friends (I'd be remiss if I called them co-workers)/patients there that I would see them on Tuesday and I did not return for months. There were medical appointments after appointments after appointments.

Our family is surrounded by love right now. We really feel it, and while I know each and every person that has reached out deserves a personal response, I haven't been able to get back to everybody yet, but I will. We are so thankful for all of you. We didn't plan to be surrounded by amazing people -- we just got so, so incredibly lucky in finding ourselves among you.

It looks like I will be starting chemotherapy very, very soon. Probably within a week or two. I'm just waiting on that appointment to place a port, to be followed by surgery in about 5 to 6 months.... radiation after that.

Looks like my 2017 is about to get worse, before it gets better, but I can't tell you how much I would appreciate any prayers you can throw our family's way. I'm not sure if it's the right thing to do, to ask for prayers. But I'm also living this year not second guessing my gut instincts. They've worked for me in the past.

I'm not doing this for sympathy, I don't need a pity party. Just the prayers will do, and any of your survivorship stories, I will take gratefully because knowledge is power, and that's where I'm starting.

In the meantime, that inner badass I have? She's almost back... I'm still conjuring her up. I know she'll be here again in just a minute. 🤍💙 I'm waiting for her here at the train station now.

PORT PLACEMENT

August 1, 2017

WAIT! Where's the GLASS of Port?

C hecking in to get that port placed - but I'm wearing these...

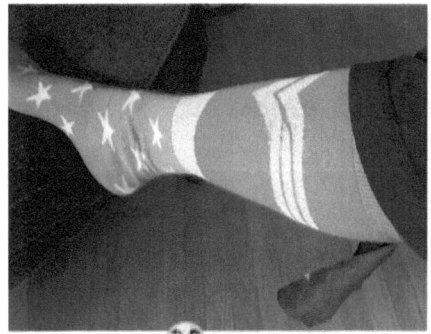

Public Service Announcement - If you ask for a "port" while you're in a hospital, you are going to be given something COMPLETELY different than what you were expecting. Be forewarned... I'm going to have to explain myself more clearly next time. 😆 My whole goal in this is to keep these kinds of miscommunications from happening to my friends. Love you guys. 🤍

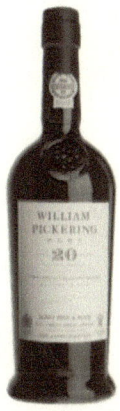

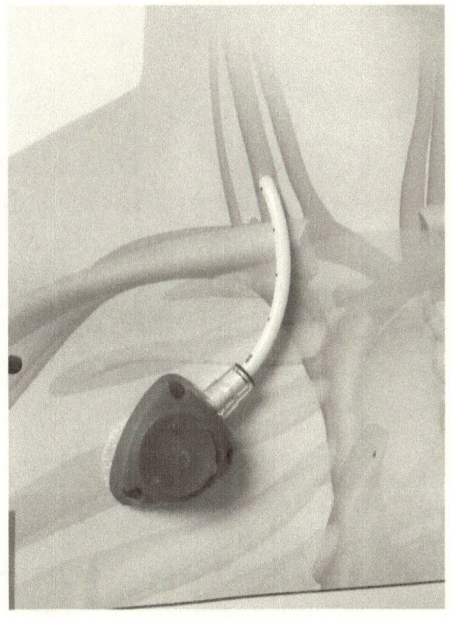

❊ ❊ ❊

CHEMOTHERAPY #1

August 2, 2017

The First Chemo? NOT so Bad...

Wonders never cease. Day One of chemo and all is well. I'm hyped up on a lot of things so they say today would go great. And it did. My mom and Tom were with me. We are watching Beauty and the Beast, family movie night. Kids were just called out to "come see the neighbors" and they CAME BACK WEARING THESE T-SHIRTS!!!

Our friends, the Pittaros, you are the best! I can't imagine what we would do without neighbors like you! Those handprints? They belong to my kids! And, my friend and neighbor Tracy, who googled, "The World's Best Lasagna" and there was such a thing -- and it lived up to it's name! Not sure what to expect in the coming days, if you don't hear right back from me... Actually, I do - I'll spare you the details. But -- you'll hear from me at some point!

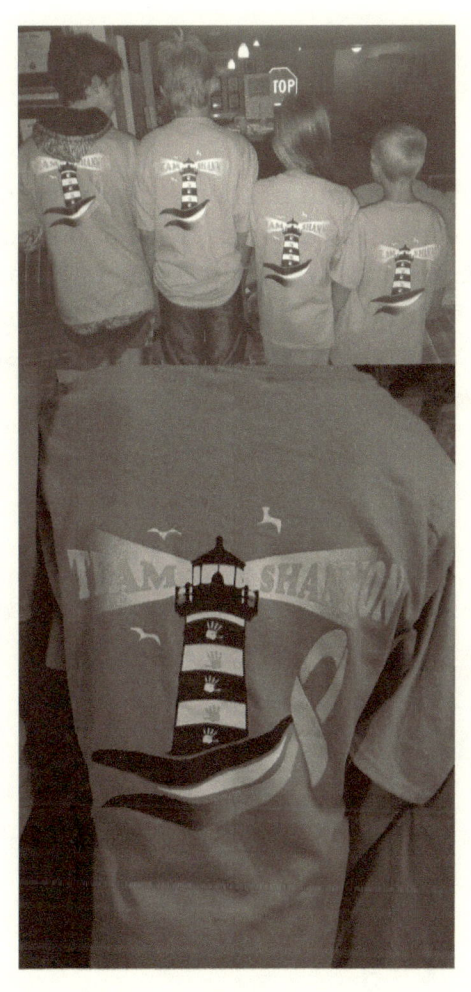

August 5, 2017

DAY 4: UGH, JUST UGH...

T he dreaded day four of chemo, round one. I haven't slept like this in years, but I'm here! Super sore, feeling not so great. But this was to be expected. And I've got some serious cuties taking care of me. Receiving everybody's good wishes, I can't believe your generosity of time, spirit and kindness... 💗🖤💗🖤💗🖤

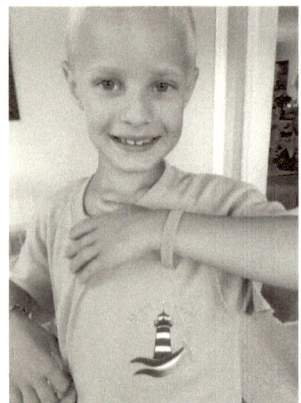

CHEMOTHERAPY #2
August 22, 2017

I ROAR IN PINK

I ROAR IN PINK. That's what my t-shirt tells me to do, so that's what I'm going to do. Chemo number two of six today. I drank the Kool-Aid when they said I might not even feel like a patient during weeks two and three. But that has not been the case. I had considered going back to work after going through round one, but I woke up every day and I asked myself if I could have gone through the motions of my day and I did not reach a yes. Days three, four and five took me out for the count. The other days leading up to day fourteen were not great either. But that beginning of week three! I suddenly woke up and felt like myself again. And it lasted all week until I lost a BUNCH of hair.

I'm actually doing something called a Dignicap. It freezes the hair follicles/scalp down to 32°, to keep the medication from entering them. It preserves your hair, although you can still lose up to 30 percent of it. Still so disconcerting to lose any.

I will have four more rounds of chemo, every three weeks. I will be moving my chemo dates to Mondays, to go through those terrible days while the kids are in school. Instead of on the weekend, like last time. Then I will wait four weeks and I will have surgery mid-December. It's going to be a long year.

Then, four weeks after that, I will start at least several weeks of daily radiation -- transfusions of immunotherapy will continue every three weeks for a year. "And that's the very latest from here!" Thank you, thank you, thank you to family, friends, neighbors and acquaintances who have extended themselves so generously, both publicly and privately. My cup runneth over. I can't even keep up with getting thank yous out to all of you, but I will.

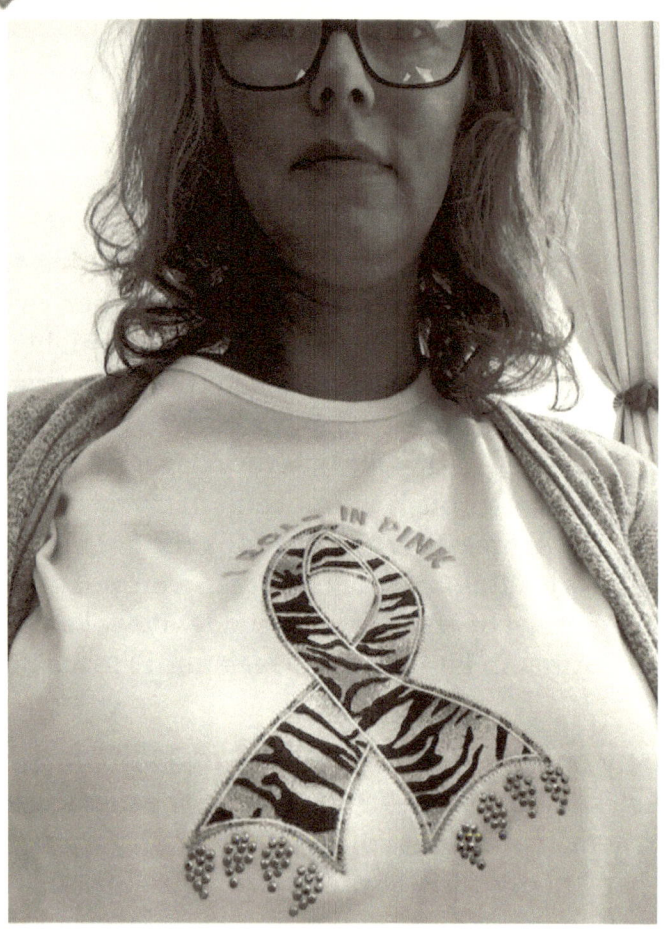

CHEMOTHERAPY #3

SEPTEMBER 11,201

Down the Rabbit Hole. Again.

"**A**nd she shall wear rings on her fingers and bells on her toes and music shall follow wherever she goes...".

Chemo #3...*sigh*...

Halfway done...but not really. I consider myself halfway done NEXT Monday, after I am past that first week. I have started describing this day as "going down the rabbit hole." I will re-surface. I don't know when; hopefully, sooner rather than later. This time I expect it to be better -- there is no fear of the unknown. The kids are back in school! And I have proverbially (and finally) picked myself up off the floor and I'm ready to fight. These two months have been extremely hard -- in my life, the worst ever.

I mourn my regular life. I miss my "crazy working mom, getting the kids to school, throwing dinner in the crockpot before I go, and looking through their school paperwork too late in the night" life. I miss my patients, I miss my desk at work, I miss my commute, even. Would you ever imagine?

23

But I realized the biggest thing I was missing the other day -- it was music. Prior to this ridiculousness, I almost always had it playing, usually singing along. So, I made a playlist -- I call it "Beast Mode". When I have it playing and I get caught up in something I love to do, I may forget for a little while, but I start getting REALLY motivated. I needed music back.

And I counted my blessings the other day when someone asked me what my pain level was. It was zero. Then they asked me how bad it was when it was at its worst. Zero. Are there symptoms of chemo? Yes, for sure. Really crappy ones. Have I been emotionally distraught? For sure. But no pain, thankfully. My immediate care plan dictates that I am two months down, ten months to go. That's why I have hesitated to ask for favors, that's why I've hesitated to take everyone up on their offers. This will be a long haul, but my cup runneth over with your good will and I thank my lucky stars every day to have crossed paths with you generous people. The gifts that have arrived at my doorstep warm my heart.

So, things I carry with me today, thanks to many of you, include:

A talisman key necklace that says "COURAGE," given to me by a cancer survivor who wore it during her treatment...

A pink "Team Shannon" bracelet...

A bangle bracelet that says "STRENGTH"...

A bangle bracelet that says "COURAGE"...

A bangle bracelet that says, "SHE BELIEVED SHE COULD, SO SHE DID"...

A headband that says, "FIERCE"...

A Healing Prayer to St. Jude prayer card...

"Our Lady of Knock" prayer card and Holy Water...

A card, "The bumblebee flies because no one told them they can't..."

A pink "Breathe Blessing" bracelet...

"Fighting Pretty" pink boxing gloves...

A Healing token...

A prayer shawl...

A Guardian angel token...

A wooden cross made of the Wye Mills, Maryland oak tree and blessed by their church...

An origami one dollar bill made into a heart...

A coin with a cross, to remind me of God's Love...

A pink beaded bracelet, with proceeds benefiting breast cancer research...

A neck pillow with a pink ribbon...

A book called "Fight On"...

And a Life is Good t-shirt that says "Namaste"...

And, of course, my Wonder Woman socks. I always wear my Wonder Woman socks.

I carry these reminders of love and grace with me to my chemotherapy appointment today. I am like a bag lady of hope, a gypsy of gratitude. I am blinged out with reminders to fight!

Whatever it takes.

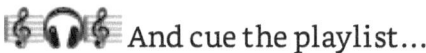 And cue the playlist...

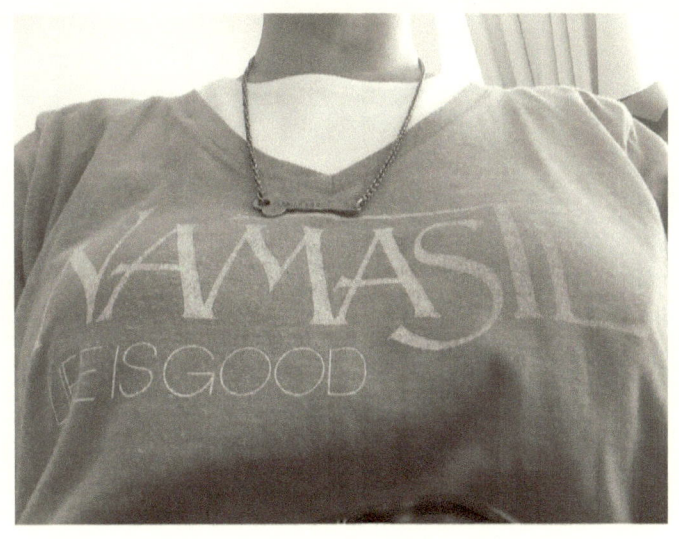

CHEMOTHERAPY #4

SURVIVOR TRAPPED IN A SEA OF PINK

And now for chemo number four out of six for those keeping score at home. Not so fun. At all. I initially planned for my posts to ease burdens on my children. I didn't want people wondering about the "strange happenings underfoot" that were happening at our house. I wanted their friends and their families to catch them if they fell.

But what I received back were blessings in spades. Your positive feedback has been amazing -- your prayers, your blessings, your gifts of generosity, your words of strength and encouragement. Your willingness to see me cry. Or maybe you didn't have a choice.

As I continued to receive more and more feedback, I started to get this sinking feeling, though, that there has not been truth in my advertising. I was talking to a friend this weekend. I said that I might not be able to post this round. That it would be too raw and emotional; I would sound petty and miserable. Maybe even vicious. I would lose friends and get unfriended! I don't want to simply complain about seemingly petty problems, especially with the recent state of world events. But she said that it's still my truth and she'd still want to hear it. So....

I have NOT acted like a "rock star," like some of you have told me. I have actually acted like a mess, the exact opposite of a rock star. I have walked into doctor's offices and the simple act of the receptionist giving me a bright, "Hello! How are you doing today?" has reduced me to exploding, leaking tears. Simply put, I'm NEVER going to be okay walking into an oncologist's office. NEVER.

And I have also taken strangers and doctor's offices employees down with me with my emotions. They end up crying along with me. They inevitably open up about their own experiences with breast cancer or cancers of other types and for a moment, I am back where I feel comfortable, if only for a moment -- that place where I can offer advice that my patients used to ask for in my real life.

Maybe they'll start to figure out my need for role reversal at some point, but I hope not. It's relevant to my happiness. A disclaimer: my EXTREMELY hormonal cancer is battled by EXTREMELY anti-hormonal ways and means. In some ways, I can't help the emotional aspects to this. In other ways? This whole thing still sucks no matter what.

And people are so kind to ask, "How are you feeling?" but the answer is not a neatly packaged gift with a bow on top. How am I feeling? I can only tell some of you, "I feel like I'm living in a f$*#ing nightmare." But that's the truth! I have symptoms that would be impolite to talk about, some would consider them to be "TMI." It's why I appreciate offers to visit, but don't really accept them too often. Drop-in guests may recognize my deer in the headlights look. I hope.

"How are you doing?" The answer is terrible -- you know I am someone who needs all of my ducks in a row. Except that NOW it feels like someone has taken all of my ducks and thrown them into the air. And added about 1000 ducks. I see the disappointment in your eyes when I give my negative, albeit truthful response. I can't say that I'm doing good, at least not yet. Maybe soon.

Each round of chemo has a cumulative effect, it took me about 12 to 14 days last time to pull out of it. It is SO frustrating. I missed my high schooler's Back to School Night. I missed my little guy's soccer game. At a cross country meet, I suddenly realized how far I was from the safety of my home. The fatigue is insane. I HAVE to be in bed most nights by 8:00.

There are days that my kids spend without solid interaction with me. I'm in bed when they leave, I'm on the couch when they get home from school, back in bed a few hours later, for several days in a row. In between it all, real life doesn't stop. The laundry needs go on, the lawn still needs to get mowed, the kids need to get to where they need to be.

Tom has taken over making school lunches in addition to breakfast duty. I haven't seen him write love notes in Sharpie on their bananas yet, but I did notice hearts drawn all over Claire's sandwich baggie the other day. Now, if I can just get him to remember some raw veggies in those lunches...

I am not used to this level of inactivity - I am used to barreling through my day at warp speed. I prefer it there.

You may have seen me this week. I was trying to SHOVE as much normal stuff into that one good week as possible -- orthodontist appointments, Cub Scout leader's meeting, Girl Scout events and we were even able to have our "Dog Pound" block party. I felt slightly closer to normal. But back down the rabbit hole again today, my loves, my friends.

I will wake up out of this "fugue state" next week to try to gather some ducks. The car needs to be inspected! It failed. Sign a kid up for the PSATs ASAP! "Mommy, when are you going to be able to come to my cross country meet? You haven't been able to make it to one yet and the other parents are there." Spirit Week this week - wear red (not everyone has a red t-shirt here), wear neon, wear sunglasses -- some days are harder than others.

In July, when I was diagnosed, I had NO idea I'd be honoring Breast Cancer Awareness in this way this month. Of COURSE, having a little girl meant that pink streaks would make it into her hair in previous years. She and I even have both donated our hair twice but, just so you know, that will NOT give you a discount on your own wig someday.

This is surely a unique place to be this October, in this month of hope. But I will embrace it. A friend from town brought a homemade wreath for the door that went straight up. I read the Wall of Hope chalkboard quotes at my Oncologist's office and I'll try to take them to heart.

Tom's immediate way of coping was to form a team to walk in the Making Strides walk on October 15th. We have no wish for people to feel uncomfortable. We KNOW that's the same exact time as our town's Education Foundation walk...and that's okay. We are happy for whatever anybody can do. We are not disappointed by what they can't. We did not expect to be in this predicament.

Finally, I have to say I've had a lot of weird things said to me during this horror show, I will include them in the book I write about this experience someday, 😀, it's going to be a dramatic comedy. But, I was told recently that I wasn't acting like a survivor. In relating this story, my friend dramatically emoted to me, "OF COURSE you are acting like a survivor!!!! You're surviving, right?? You survived today? Then you're a SURVIVOR, for gosh sakes!!" There were some swear words I left out to protect the innocent. 😀Here are the lyrics to one of the songs on my Beast Mode playlist. Do yourself a favor and give it a listen to today. You'll be better for it: Survivor by Destiny's Child. After that, go back to the Foo Fighters for the rest of the day. 😎 And I will keep on surviving over here. With my Wonder Woman socks on.

Now that you're out of my life, I'm so much better

You thought that I'd be weak without you, but I'm stronger

You thought that I'd be broke without you, but I'm richer

You thought that I'd be sad without you, I laugh harder

Thought I wouldn't grow without you, now I'm wiser

Thought that I'd be helpless without you, but I'm smarter

You thought that I'd be stressed without you, but I'm chillin'

You thought I wouldn't sell without you, sold nine million

I'm a survivor (what?)

I'm not gon' give up (what?)

I'm not gon' stop (what?)

I'm gon' work harder (what?)

I'm a survivor (what?)

I'm gonna make it (what?)

I will survive (what?)

Keep on survivin'(what?)

WALL OF HOPE
WORDS OF COURAGE & STRENGTH.
FALL DOWN
BLESSINGS!
LIVE
LOVE
LAUGH
tough times
NEVER LAST...
By His Stripes

HOPE

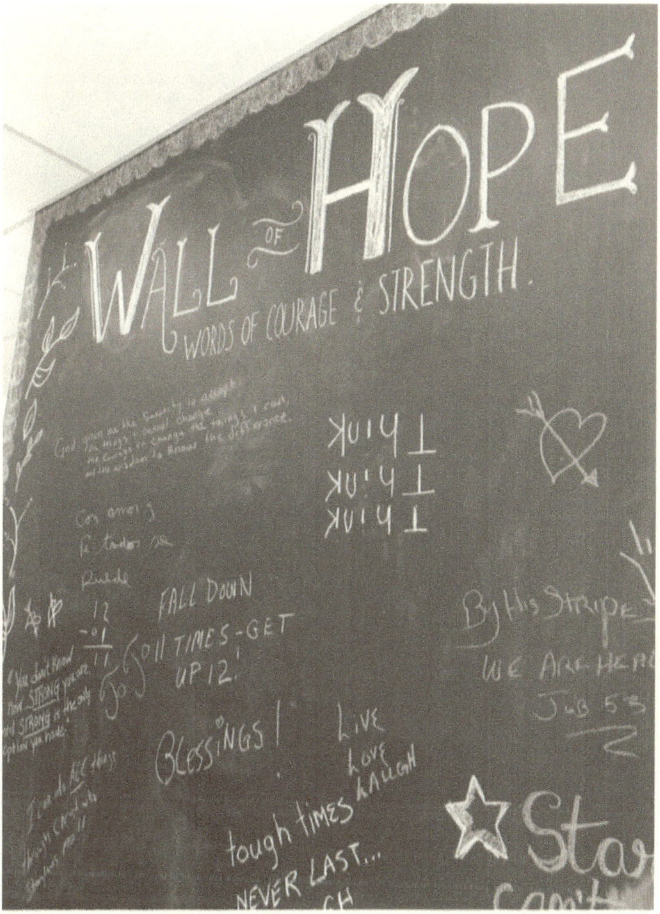

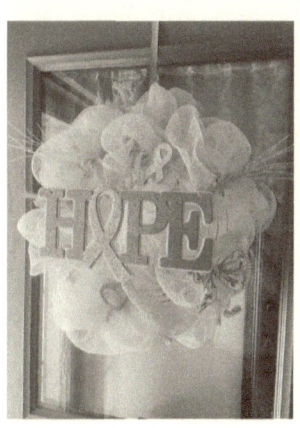

Dr. Shannon M. Mulvey

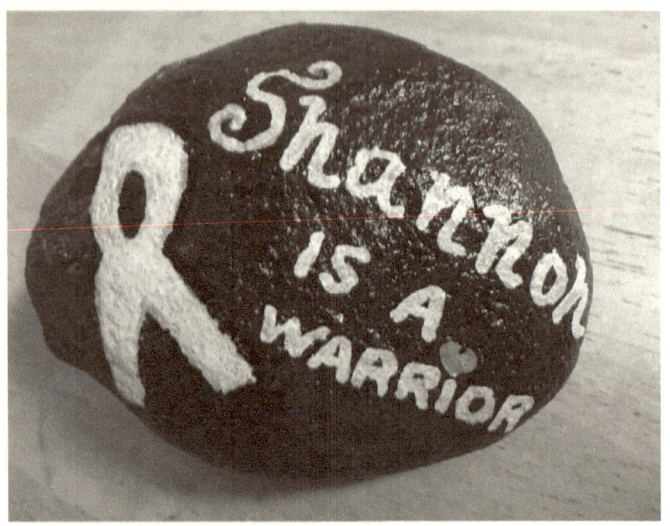

* * *

"THE WALK"

October 15, 2017
My Cup Runneth Over

Another shout out to all of my amazing team members walking on Sunday morning! When Tom made this team, I knew it was his way of coping with this ridiculousness. I never expected to walk with anybody other than my family. I can't believe the response from our team members that signed up to walk with us. My cup runneth over. Love you guys. And thanks to those that will be wearing their Team Shannon T-shirts even if they can't be with us physically and to those that donated.

Walking with my team... 🖤🖤🖤

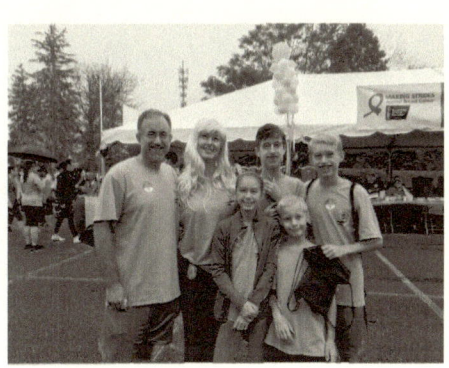

Dr. Shannon M. Mulvey

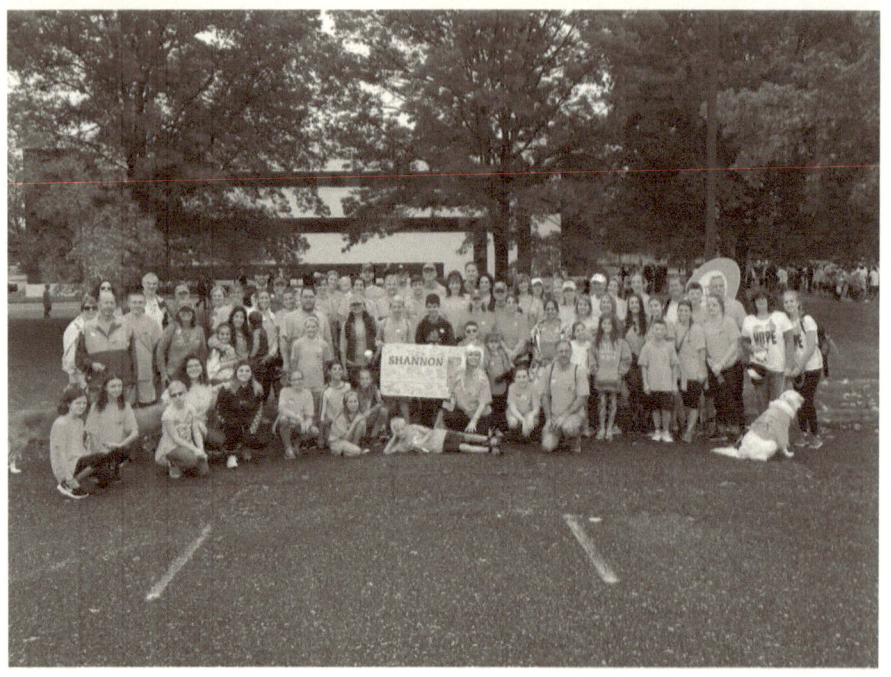

CHEMOTHERAPY #5

OCTOBER 23, 2017

THRIVING

If you're playing along at home, today is chemo number five out of six. Of course I'm wearing my Wonder Woman socks. Sounds like significant progress, right? Mostly to me, too. I can't tell you how I am HOLDING on to being done with this part of the mess within the month. Chemo today and then again three weeks from today. Grant me an extra week from there. And in the (to me) now immortal words of a certain Julia Louis Dreyfus, "Chemo #5: finito. We are NOT fucking around here." I couldn't say it any better myself. Let the plagiarism and the sentiment stand. Because I concur.

And I'd like to make a Public Service Announcement: the new quest for attainment is to be a "Thriver," not JUST a "Survivor". I learned that as a guest of St. Barnabas' Fashion for the Pink Crusade event on Wednesday night. I haven't been able to let that word go. I took that goal with me, as I did the incredible stories I heard from the Survivors AND the Thrivers that were there. Beautiful, beautiful women and their sentiments.

October brought a lot of milestones to me, some good, some frustrating. It turns out that it has NOT been easy to be a somewhat newly diagnosed breast cancer patient smack dab in the middle of Breast Cancer Awareness month. There are some benefits. People are so kind to remember me at this time.

And there are the scary moments -- simply turning on the Today show may bring you a beautiful woman fighting (and thriving) during her battle, so inspiring, but you may also get a family's follow-up story, from the previous year, of the beautiful family she has now left behind..."but what a legacy she left." Losing Michelle Marsh at age 63 to breast cancer this week, too young. Julia Louis Dreyfus throwing her hat into the ring as a "1 in 8er" both gave me hope and also bothered me as she appears to be the epitome of health. You hear about Olivia Newton John's cancer returning and how it felt for Shannon Doherty to lose her hair. It's everywhere to me.

Tucking Max in the other night, he asked me, "Mommy, did you ever know somebody who died of breast cancer?" That was followed up by, "How did you get breast cancer?" You can't practice for those conversations. And it turns out that Claire didn't actually know what a mastectomy was, despite this word being thrown around. I am an AVID pro-breastfeeder, my kids know that about me. It must have been shocking to a prepubescent tween to hear what the surgery would actually accomplish.

Another milestone I hit this month was the three month anniversary of my diagnosis. It has ONLY been three months -- why am I expecting to have processed this? Why are others expecting me to have processed this? I don't get frustrated by it, just perplexed.

Just like Forrest Gump decides he will stop running after his jog turns into a three-year, two-month, 14-day and 16-hour crisscross of the entire United States with an, "I'm pretty tired. I think I'll go home now," I do believe that my crying is finally done now. I can hear the collective sigh of relief. I feel it from myself, too. Remember the part about it being a hormonal cancer. These tears have LEAKED out of me, uninvited. At least for now, I've reached the bottom of the well, it seems.

Another milestone -- I walked the Breast Cancer walk for the first time, with my family and 75 of my besties. They came from Florida, Maryland, there were babes in strollers, three dogs and a couple of peeps there with hangovers (I won't out them). My Girl Scouts were there, my Cub Scouts, Boy Scouts, Sam even ran it, despite getting four wisdom teeth removed three days prior.

The shirts were amazing and, in typical Susan fashion (they just KNOW things) having blue shirts to wear in a sea of pink proved fortuitous. I never had any problem linking up to my teammates I found along the way.

I wore my wigs for the first time this month. I wore a pink one for the walk, I loved it. It was sent home by Tom's co-workers for the occasion. The only monkey wrench was when Tom thought it was for HIM. I don't know, aren't middle aged men supposed to embrace their bald spots? Middle aged women should be given a couple of options before deciding to embrace theirs. I was shocked to discover that this Five Below wig stayed on better than the real wig I purchased, which I have now also worn for the first time.

I guess I would have to actually go on Twitter to start a Twitter war, but when I learned this week that my insurance company would not cover the wig, I started composing Tweets in my head about this further evidence of insurance company fleecing. "Dear Insurance Company, It is with great displeasure that I discover that you do not cover wigs for your cancer patients. I consider that bad business. Strangely, after behind on hold for almost two hours, it is also a shock that I don't qualify for your cancer program either. You can go back to playing golf now at the five-star resort you flew yourself and your top producers to to congratulate yourself on saving THAT money. Phew -- I am SURE that was a close one, right? Order a double Scotch on the rocks, you'll be all right in a few..." I know that's more than 180 characters, by the way.

Being out at a fashion show was a fun night out this week and being surrounded by these thriving ladies inspired me and made me ALMOST feel normal.

A very favorite teacher of my children entered into her own battle this month. Another mom in town confided to me her own diagnosis. These stories have brought me incredible sadness but I also believe have helped pull me out of the abyss. I have put the proverbial oxygen mask on myself to now mentor them through their journey as a friend has taken on mentoring me. I have seen THREE ten-year survivors celebrating their survivor/thrivership this month and that's what I am aiming for. There are a lot of us!

So, chemo is almost done. Mastectomy in December. Still trying to wrap my head around THAT one...but one ridiculousness at a time.

A friend from town sent a card that related, and I wish I had the quote exactly right, to make sure I handle this cancer diagnosis MY way -- even if it means crying, screaming or dancing in the street. I love that. Join in if you see me. I'll be wearing my Wonder Woman socks.

And, in any case, the Foo Fighters just (finally) announced their NYC shows for 2018 while I've been composing this, so I have to go now. Tom needs me to help plan the details of getting us there. More proof that things will start looking up soon.

Foo Fighters - Best of You

*I've got another confession to make * I'm your fool * Everyone's got their chains to break * Holdin' you **

*Were you born to resist or be abused? **

*Is someone getting the best, the best, the best, the best of you? * Is someone getting the best, the best, the best, the best of you? **

*Are you gone and onto someone new? * I needed somewhere to hang my head * Without your noose * You gave me something that I didn't have * But had no use * I was too weak to give in * Too strong to lose * My heart is under arrest again * But I break loose * My head is giving me life or death * But I can't choose * I swear I'll never give in * I refuse **

*Has someone taken your faith? * Its real, the pain you feel* You trust, you must * Confess * Is someone getting the best, the best, the best, the best of you? **

*Has someone taken your faith? * Its real, the pain you feel * The life, the love * You die to heal * The hope that starts * The broken hearts * You trust, you must * Confess*

*Is someone getting the best, the best, the best, the best of you? * Is someone getting the best, the best, the best, the best of you?*

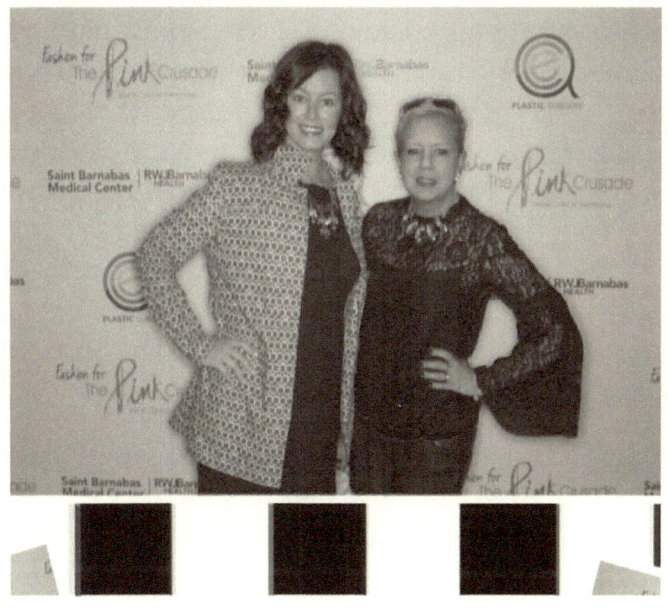

CHEMOTHERAPY #6

NOVEMBER 13, 2017

Chop? Cut? Rip? We're Not in the Kitchen!!

C hemo number six today. Of six. I'm all hooked up, my head is frozen down to a balmy 32 degrees. Tom is here. For a little while, I have to pretend that it's not poison dripping into my system and that it's a life-saving cure. My platelets are really low today. They had to adjust some of the chemo drug percentages, otherwise I was going to have to wait until next week. Since I have to have surgery four weeks later, this already brings us to 12/12. So I'm glad that I don't have to wait a week longer for that. Getting through the Christmas holidays is going to be hard enough this year.

In one of my last chemo posts, I included the lyrics to Foo Fighters "Best of You." It's in my Beast Mode playlist for battling this specter in my house. As Tom and I got in the car this morning, it was playing. A fantastic harbinger of great things to come. It was a good sign to me!

As happy as I am to be starting my last chemo today, it does bring about a certain feeling of a post traumatic stress disorder response. I know the next 10 to 12 days will be arduous. The cumulative effect of the chemo has caught up with me. I have gotten into bed as early as 6:30 or 7:00 on some nights. I have missed track meets, trick-or-treating with my children, there's been a bunch of breakfasts for dinner. But the kids have been flexible, maybe even thankful, for too much screen time.

Since my diagnosis, I have learned of three more women I know chosen to fight this battle. It feels like it's an epidemic! This last chemo definitely closes a certain Stranger Things chapter in my autumn. Just give me one more week on the couch AND the last four episodes of season two.

My new chapter opens up with words I hear like this:

"You should chop them off. I would."

"You should get rid of those puppies."

"Look at it this way, now you'll have a nice pair of perky cheerleader ----."

"Of course you should take both off. Do you really want one 36 wide and one 36 long?"

"This treatment will push you into menopause. But you're 45, so that's OK."

Well, that's not okay to me.

I shared a link last week, "Things not to say to breast cancer patients." When I read some of the comments, I agreed with them. I know that people are doing their best, I know that people don't know what to say. I appreciate all of them! Unfortunately, the above statements that people have conveyed to me were not included in that article.

My dilemma is that the cancer has only presented in one breast. I do not carry the gene, I have no family history and no risk factors. I have to chalk this up to a random act of violence in this left breast of mine. Current research shows that there is only a one to three percent chance of it presenting in the other breast.

It is much more likely to go to an organ or the bones or the brain.

And in our horrifyingly disposable society. it becomes a "let's just throw it out, just in case." People just opt for it to go. This particularly happens in America. When I think of a lung cancer patient, with the cancer presenting in one lung -- would you get rid of the other lung? No! It's quite the conundrum.

In more silly news, when in the midst of a general conversation, when I turn away for a moment, as typically happens during the course of a normal conversation, sometimes when I turn back, I catch my co-conversationalist sneaking a peek to see if they can figure out which breast it is...ha ha ha! It can NOT be seen with the naked eye! This strikes me as funny.

Most people close to me know I almost exclusively voice text. If I had to type out texts, no one would ever hear from me again. So, occasionally something escapes into the cyberworld if I don't proofread it before I hit send. A silly thing that happens is that it changes one of my children's names to the word "sex." It is very uncomfortable when I realize that I have just sent a text to a friend that says something like, "I am at the school looking for sex." That is NOT THE TRUTH.

But the word "mastectomy," as translated by my voice texts, usually translates to "mystic to me" and, in typical art imitates life fashion, this whole thing IS mystical to me. I am particularly affected right now by this #METOO sensation sweeping insidiously across the country. It seems to be a very cookie-cutter recipe. Men in power, taking advantage of less advantaged women (and in some cases men and children), without a care for their wellbeing.

What does this have to do with the above statements? The statements to me were made by women. I am not a wordsmith, but this vocabulary that women use against themselves is violent in my eyes. Chop off, rip off, cut off often because you are done using them for babies. But does that mean they're useless after children? They still have function.

Do men "chop off" their private parts when they're done having children? Would someone suggest that they do that? This is not meant to start a larger debate, it's just thoughts that go through my head while trying to make this very personal and very nerve wracking decision. Women have to be better to themselves to stand up to these David and Goliath circumstances in which we sometimes find ourselves.

As part of my natural childbirth teachings, I used to talk about America's very Puritanical roots. We still have these very Pilgrim-like traditions in our heads. It is why a woman with exposed breasts inspires a Beavis and Butthead response from a stranger and a mother nursing her baby might be considered disgusting by some. And so a diseased breast has to go, but our society thinks nothing of taking the other one, too. This does not apply to those people who have tested positive for the gene.

Eventually, you do have this surgery and there have to be a lot of benefits to looking like you looked before, clothes fitting like they fit before and feeling a lot closer to normal then you've been in a while. But we cross the line to danger when we are just putting them back on to look more desirable to others because they don't return to you with function.

Sense of self has to come from what YOU think of yourself, not what others think of you. Isn't that what we teach our children? I still have not made this decision yet; I will probably use up every minute, right until go time, trying to figure this ONE out. It's a tough one and I don't think you can make the decision if you are not the one stuck in this tornado.

I have learned this year that no matter what kind of cancer presents to you or your family, it comes with massive amounts of losses. There are the "little things" that people tell you aren't important right now. The house is not getting cleaned like it should; and there is dismal progress on my type A "to do" list. How will Christmas proceed with the traditions that are important to my children?

Losses also include little things like my eyebrows and eyelashes. I miss them when I look in the mirror. Now I'm obsessed with all of yours! You all look like you have fuzzy caterpillars on top of your eyes and I mean that in the best possible of ways. Claire and Max miss that we don't have any capers in the fridge. They BOTH have asked for some this week. The fridge isn't stocked like it would usually be.

I miss my stamina almost the most. I did a five-mile hike in Harriman State Park this time last year with my family. That is not even a remote possibility at this point.

I miss my hormones. The estrogen that they are trying to street fight out of me has a heart protective factor. We have heart disease in my family and have had two family members not survive heart attacks. I thought my estrogen would be so useful for battling that.

I'm REALLY going to miss this left breast. I've been good to it, even though it tried to kill me. I sleep on my left side, I expected it to support me for years to come. But, out of all of the things I would miss the most, it would have to be my right breast. Because that one has been very unassuming and was just hanging around, doing what it was supposed to be doing, being a good listener.

Four weeks from tomorrow, I will have made this decision. But it won't come easy. As I end this post, both chemo drugs are out of my IV drip - a very, very significant moment. Just waiting on my two immunotherapy drugs to make their way through now. Wearing my Wonder Woman socks. 🤍🖤

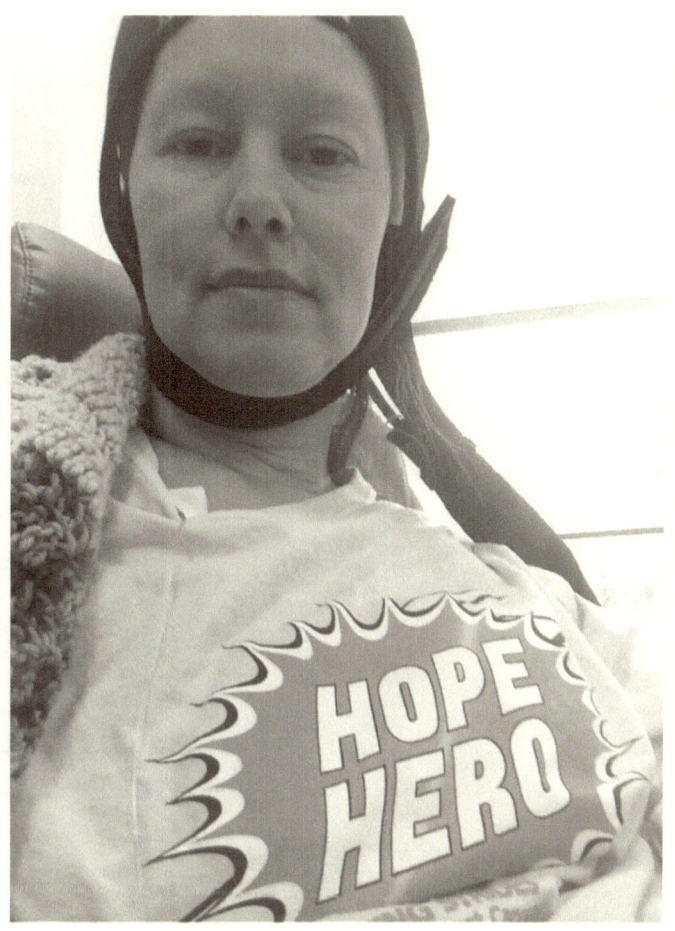

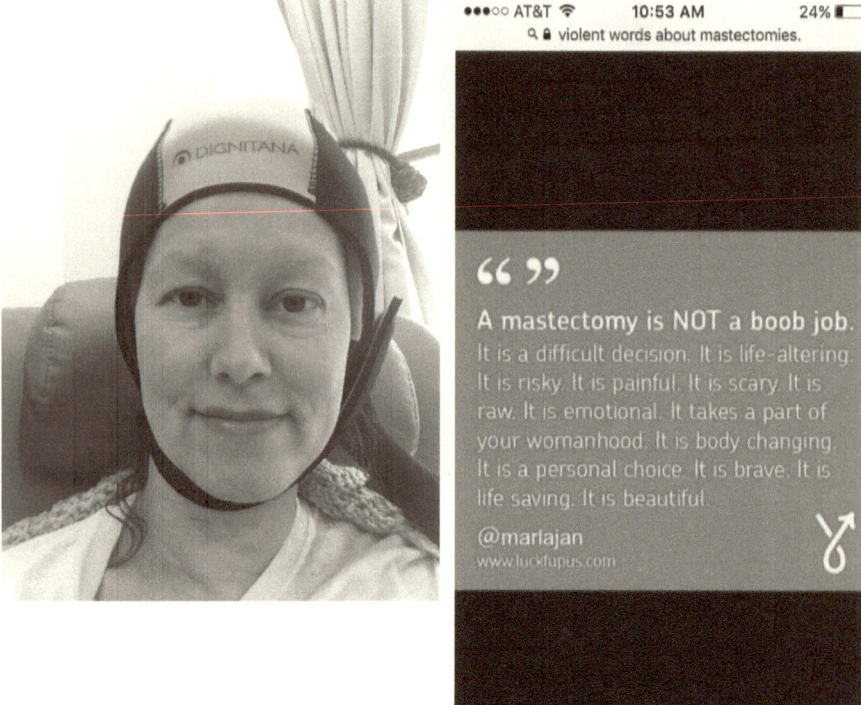

MONOCLONAL ANTIBODIES INFUSIONS

DECEMBER 4, 2017

NOT SICK BUT STRONG

"Not sick but strong."

This is where I derive my motivation from today. I am BACK in "the chair." But there will be no chemo drugs coming through my port today. Instead? There will be "monoclonal antibodies." These are the ingredients in the cocktail that need to be infused every three weeks until next fall.

But I am beyond thankful to not have those chemo symptoms this week. And, instead of a five- or six-hour "stay," it will only be an hour or two. So I expect this post to be shorter than usual, but making these posts are how I get my mind off what is actually happening. I guess if I was an artist, I would be painting away.

I had even more to be thankful for this Thanksgiving. I received the news that the chemo appears to be working. Long exhale...

The follow-up mammogram, ultrasound and breast MRI yielded this news: I have had a "tremendous response" to chemotherapy and "near complete resolution." Previously noted chest wall enhancement is no longer seen. She said I should celebrate, not everybody gets this kind of response. Everything continues as scheduled -- surgery, radiation, transfusions for a year. But what an unbelievable Thanksgiving present this year.

In the meantime, I am scheduled for surgery one week from tomorrow. Many people have asked if I am nervous. I am not. I am sad about it. This is SUCH an emotional journey, and beyond difficult to be doing this two weeks before Christmas. So much has been taken off the proverbial list. No Christmas cards this year. To trudge into see that Rockefeller tree is also off the list. I have very little stamina right now. Even a flight of stairs proves difficult. But it appears I will get more time to sit by the Christmas tree lights and who doesn't wish for more of that during the magic of the season? I DID get the kids to get that picture with Santa -- that was quite the feat! My kids are good sports.

My Claire -- she is an AVID mythology fan. I wish there was a stronger word than avid. I wouldn't want to use the word obsessive, but her excitement is close to that (towards Hamilton, too. Her brothers have decided that they hate Hamilton because of her near constant singing [rapping?] of the lyrics).

She can name all of the gods, the mythological creatures, whether it is a Greek god, a Roman god, a Norse god and all of their background stories. Her one birthday present request last August was for a bow and arrow. "And though she be but little, she is fierce."

But Claire gets upset when she sees me upset and there is no manual on how to handle this. She wrapped her arms around me the other night and told me about the book she just read. It came off the classroom bookshelf, but it happened to be about a young girl and her mother, who has just been diagnosed with breast cancer. In Claire's effort to lift my spirits, she related something she learned.

She said that Amazon women, in an effort to become better

archers, willingly removed a breast. "They volunteered to do this and it made them stronger." This factoid has really gotten me thinking. Wonder Woman has been a recurring theme in my battle with breast cancer. I have received cards, stickers and analogies of her. It turns out, and to come full circle for non-comic strip fans, that Wonder Woman was the only daughter of an Amazon queen! Later renditions have her as the daughter of Zeus. But those Amazon women -- how FIERCE!

I wouldn't willingly sign up for this ridiculousness; I'd advise against it, too, but I will continue to Amazon this out, Wonder Woman this out and hope to make my family proud. I don't know if I will take up archery, but it appears I will have the advantage, if I choose to become an archer. Who knew? When one door closes, another one opens.

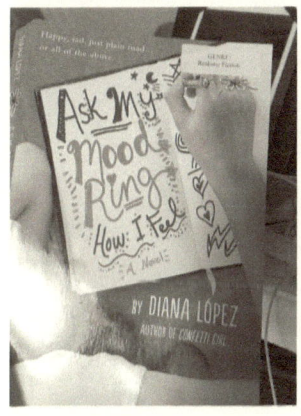

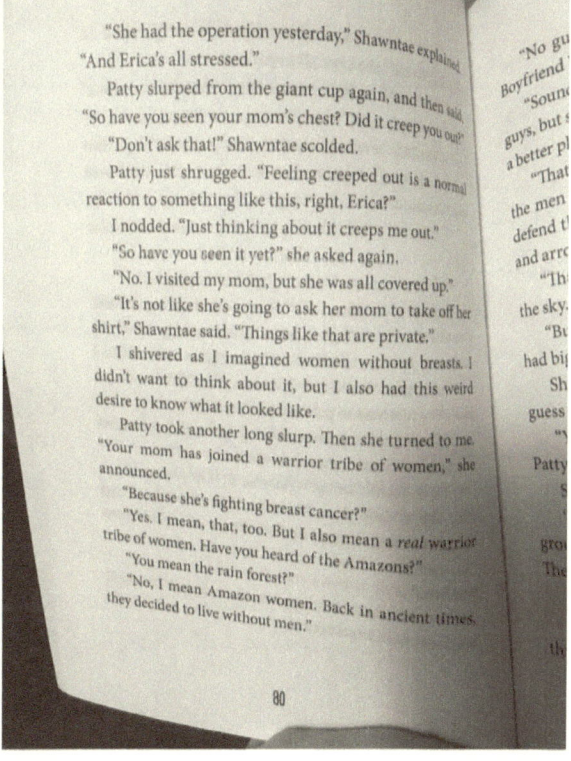

"She had the operation yesterday," Shawntae explained. "And Erica's all stressed."

Patty slurped from the giant cup again, and then said, "So have you seen your mom's chest? Did it creep you out?"

"Don't ask that!" Shawntae scolded.

Patty just shrugged. "Feeling creeped out is a normal reaction to something like this, right, Erica?"

I nodded. "Just thinking about it creeps me out."

"So have you seen it yet?" she asked again.

"No. I visited my mom, but she was all covered up."

"It's not like she's going to ask her mom to take off her shirt," Shawntae said. "Things like that are private."

I shivered as I imagined women without breasts. I didn't want to think about it, but I also had this weird desire to know what it looked like.

Patty took another long slurp. Then she turned to me. "Your mom has joined a warrior tribe of women," she announced.

"Because she's fighting breast cancer?"

"Yes. I mean, that, too. But I also mean a *real* warrior tribe of women. Have you heard of the Amazons?"

"You mean the rain forest?"

"No, I mean Amazon women. Back in ancient times, they decided to live without men."

80

"She had the operation yesterday," Shawntae explained. "And Erica's all stressed."

Patty slurped from the giant cup again, and then said, "So have you seen your mom's chest? Did it creep you out?"

"Don't ask that!" Shawntae scolded.

Patty just shrugged. "Feeling creeped out is a normal reaction to something like this, right, Erica?"

I nodded. "Just thinking about it creeps me out."

"So have you seen it yet?" she asked again.

"No. I visited my mom, but she was all covered up."

"It's not like she's going to ask her mom to take off her shirt," Shawntae said. "Things like that are private."

I shivered as I imagined women without breasts. I didn't want to think about it, but I also had this weird desire to know what it looked like.

Patty took another long slurp. Then she turned to me.

"Your mom has joined a warrior tribe of women," she announced.

"Because she's fighting breast cancer?"

"Yes, I mean, that, too. But I also mean a real warrior tribe of women. Have you heard of the Amazons?"

"You mean the rain forest?"

"No, I mean Amazon women. Back in ancient times, they decided to live without men."

"No guys?" I felt scandalized. How could you have a Boyfriend Wish List when there weren't any guys around?

"Sounds like a good idea to me," Shawntae said. "I like guys but sometimes they're overrated. This world would be a better place with more women as mayors and presidents."

"That's what the Amazons thought," Patty said. "But the men kept trying to take over. So they had to learn to defend themselves, and their favorite weapon was the bow and arrow."

"That's cool," I said, imagining arrows arcing across the sky.

"But there was a problem," Patty added. "The Amazons had big breasts that got in the way."

Shawntae stood up, pretended to pull back on a bow. "I guess it'd be hard if you had giant boobs."

"You want to know how they solved the problem?" Patty asked.

Shawntae and I nodded.

"They cut off the breast. Can you imagine a whole group of women walking around like that? But it worked. They were the best archers around."

"They weren't sick?" I asked.

"No, they weren't sick at all. They volunteered to do this, and it made them stronger."

I imagined a tribe of women warriors in the forest. They had long hair, muscular arms and legs, and white tunics. One side flat. But they were wrestling, swimming, and running through obstacle courses. And mom was with them, doing all of those things -- not sick but strong.

Excerpt taken from *Ask My Mood Ring How I Feel*, by Diana Lopez.

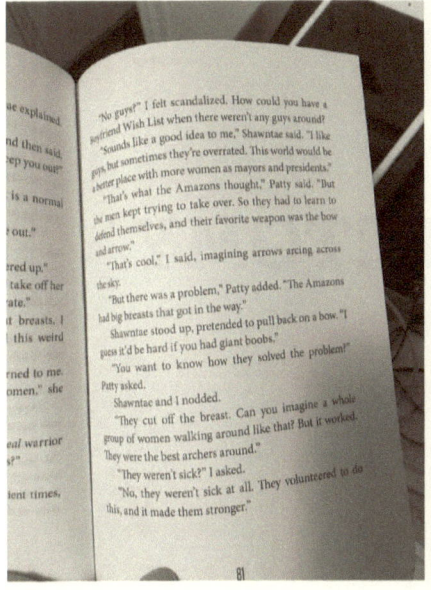

e explained.

nd then said,
eep you out?"

is a normal

e out."

ered up."
take off her
ate."
t breasts. I
this weird

rned to me.
omen," she

eal warrior
?"

ient times,

"No guys!" I felt scandalized. How could you have a boyfriend Wish List when there weren't any guys around?

"Sounds like a good idea to me," Shawntae said. "I like guys, but sometimes they're overrated. This world would be a better place with more women as mayors and presidents."

"That's what the Amazons thought," Patty said. "But the men kept trying to take over. So they had to learn to defend themselves, and their favorite weapon was the bow and arrow."

"That's cool," I said, imagining arrows arcing across the sky.

"But there was a problem," Patty added. "The Amazons had big breasts that got in the way."

Shawntae stood up, pretended to pull back on a bow. "I guess it'd be hard if you had giant boobs."

"You want to know how they solved the problem?" Patty asked.

Shawntae and I nodded.

"They cut off the breast. Can you imagine a whole group of women walking around like that? But it worked. They were the best archers around."

"They weren't sick?" I asked.

"No, they weren't sick at all. They volunteered to do this, and it made them stronger."

81

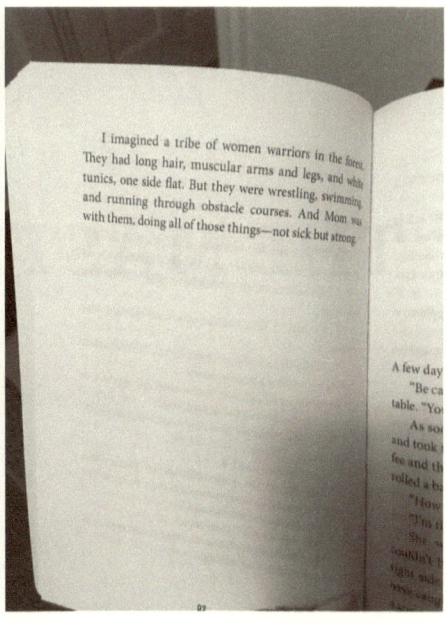

I imagined a tribe of women warriors in the forest. They had long hair, muscular arms and legs, and white tunics, one side flat. But they were wrestling, swimming, and running through obstacle courses. And Mom was with them, doing all of those things—not sick but strong.

A few day

"Be ca
table. "Yo

As so
and took
fee and th
rolled a b

"How
"I'm t
She
ouldn't
ght mile

THE MASTECTOMY

December 12, 2017

One Last Look

"O ne last look". Not an easy day -- mastectomy day. It was hard not to take a backwards glance, like leaving a loved one at the airport. In fact, it was hard not to take a few last looks. Taking a "mental picture," if you will. I have no wish to go back to the bikini days, but I still would not have wanted to change my body's lifetime of familiarity. I'm used to seeing me and now I will have to get used to a new normal. It's hard not to be angry with that left breast of mine. I was good to it. I took care of it. But it betrayed me, so now it's time to go. Farewell, my old, former friend. It is stunningly, maddeningly, crushingly bittersweet to see you go.

I will be anxious to hear the results. A radioactive tracer will be injected on the highway to unknown lymph lands. I'm hoping it finds itself on a dead end street. Hopefully, the neoadjuvant chemotherapy shrunk these imposters down into oblivion.

The surgery is expected to take two hours; the recovery about the same.

Max asked me last night when all of this will be over. This journey began 7/7/17. We have now made it to 12/12/17. Chemo is done, surgery will be done today. Radiation will begin in about a month. I am eager to close out 2017, but I am not yet done with this journey. I'm not even halfway done. That was hard to convey to him. They have put up with a lot this year. There have been a lot of tears, kisses and hugs in our house this week.

Thankfully, I had an epiphany yesterday afternoon -- after today's surgery, the cancer will be out of me. That's the goal of this therapeutic surgery. I have faith in that goal and I am working mentally towards that goal, too. But, man, it still won't make those first showers easy or that first trip to the beach.

Claire said, through tears the other night, "Mommy, you will still look beautiful to me." Out of the mouths of babes. It is so hard to take something off the outside of you. Believe me, I didn't do this for my appendix that failed me ten years ago. I don't even think about that bad boy!

Something I have to work on, and I want to interview my friends and family who have navigated these harrowing waters before me, is how in the HELL do you ever get rid of the feeling that you're waiting for the other shoe to drop? This diagnosis of mine BLEW me out of the water.

I have said that if I had been hit by a bus that day, it would not have felt any different. I guess it's a form of posttraumatic stress disorder. The person who has gotten into a car accident must deal with this when they get back into a car. The cancer patient, permit me to say victim, must always be struggling to not let themself keep looking in the rear view mirror.

I'm getting prepped for surgery now. I just had to take my Wonder Woman socks off, but I have them close and I will be looking to get them back on as soon as possible. There are doctors and nurses walking around, checking in on pre-operative patients. A nurse is giving out butterfly Christmas ornaments to her co-workers. They are handmade by her. She just said to me, "Here, take one!" I held it in my hand, I'm looking down on it. It's pretty. A social worker that I've met here was sitting with me. She just said, "Wow! Isn't that incredible? Butterflies represent metamorphosis, a change into beauty, new life. That's SO significant that you just got this!" It was hard to say goodbye to Tom. He was crying, too. He laid his head down next to mine and just held on as they started to wheel me away. This is heart wrenching.

And I have made my decision. It will be a left simple mastectomy.

I am attaching the very best devotion I could have read today...hopefully, you will grab some meaning from it, too... And, a special, special thank you to ALL of the special well wishes I woke up to today -- you guys have been carrying me through this and I appreciate you all. You're the BEST.

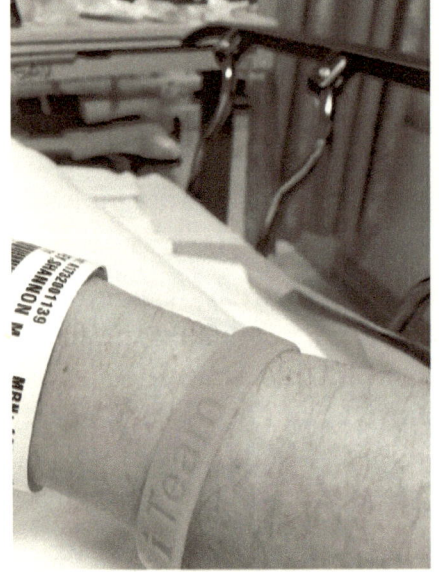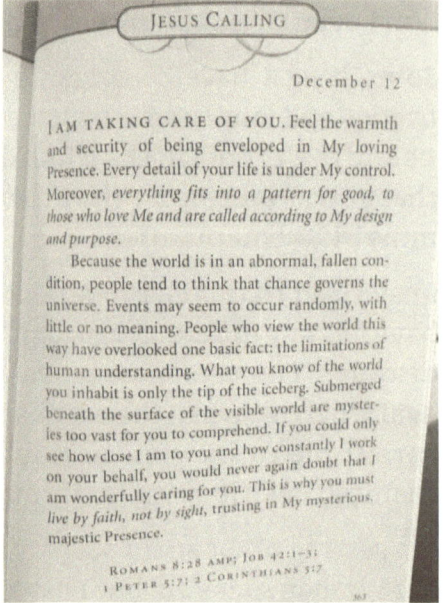

Devotion taken from Sarah Young's *Jesus Calling.*

POST-MASTECTOMY

December 19, 2017
No Words

T he drains and hoses are out! Phew! The pathology report is back. This is surely great news -- there was some residual cancer left over, according to the pathology report, but the neoadjuvant chemotherapy, along with the immuno-therapy, has done "tremendous" work. That is the adjective used. In fact, nuclear testing immediately before the surgery could not even find the sentinel node, the node which would have been first affected by breast cancer cells attempting to commute. The surgeon couldn't find it either. So, she grabbed what turned out to be a "handful" of lymph nodes. The amount grabbed was unknown until the pathology report made it clear.

Turns out there were 13 taken. Thirteen STERILE lymph nodes. Which means there HAD been cancer in at least some of them. And now there's not. Hallelujah! It is assumed, hoped, prayed for, that the residual cancer leftover was scooped up in the surgery.

And if for some reason there are STILL lurkers? Radiation, a year of transfusions and anti-estrogen pills are coming for me. It's a

LONG haul, and throw in physical therapy to combat lymphedema. We're past the first couple of chapters, but I think those were the hardest. Onward and upward.

This news was delivered with such joy yesterday. The surgeon, the nurse practitioner, the nurse -- they were SO pleased. They said I should celebrate this season! I know I will. I AM happy, I feel like I've been waiting to exhale and I was able to yesterday. The news was also delivered that I dropped from stage 3B to stage 2B.

So, why didn't I have this overwhelming display of emotion and why didn't I get all slobbery like the situation may have dictated? Why didn't the passionate, dramatic music start playing to a crescendo, like in a Hollywood drama? Because the well was dry. I intimated last week just how incredibly difficult that last shower was before surgery. Well, that difficulty paled in comparison to that first shower, post surgery.

My mom stayed with me for several days. She was leaving on Friday but wanted to make sure I took that first shower first. And I know why she wanted me to take it before she left. Is it needless to say? I ended up on the couch, under the covers, staring at the Christmas tree for the rest of the day. That was a mindblowingly sad day. It felt like I had been through something barbaric.

Yet, there was another reason why it was difficult to conjure up joy yesterday. It's because it's impossible to hear words like "your cancer isn't as bad anymore," without hearing the words "your cancer." I compare this whole thing to an assault that you didn't see coming. How do you get back to that massively underrated feeling of safety? I WILL get there. This is not about bravery. It's about not having a choice. Everybody would do it, given similar circumstances. There is NO CHOICE. But I'm still working through the journey.

I came across a particularly (extremely) brave woman battling her own case of breast cancer. She is astounding. She is brave. Her name is Shelly Melton. She is someone I hold before me for

59

hope. Her message reads:

> This is breast cancer.
>
> It isn't pink ribbons
>
> or sparkle "Save the tatas"
>
> It is profound loss
>
> And fear
>
> And discovery
>
> And strength
>
> And
>
> FIERCE.
>
> And I concur.

In OTHER news, I lost 8 pounds since the surgery. Just how heavy was that thing????

I AM SO happy that all the doctors seem to go on vacation this coming week. So I can take a break from this journey, too. All of my next appointments are after the new year. Happy, happy holidays to everyone! The outreach of your support has been nothing short of amazing. I still can't believe it. My family and I will forever be touched by your generosity of time, spirit and gifts. This Christmas season, I will remember each and every one of you with love and thankfulness. And in the new year, I will work very, very hard to pay it forward. I look forward to kicking 2017 in the ass now and getting to 2018 as fast as possible! See you there!

Dr. Shannon M. Mulvey

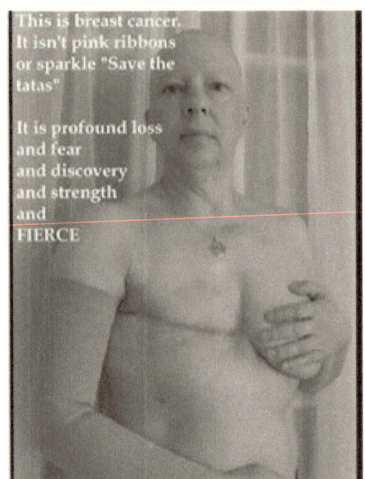

About this article

NEWS-LEADER.COM

Springfield woman, breast cancer patient, shares photo with message

Shelly Melton's brave photo of her battle with breast cancer echoes the ugly truth many face.

INFUSIONS

December 26, 2017
Every Three Weeks

I nfusion #8 out of 18. The game I'm playing every three weeks in 2018. I'm not going to write on and on about it for once. I've bored you all enough this year.

But, I can say this -- chemo symptoms are almost out of here, but not gone quite yet and I'm glad to be two weeks past the surgery. That part is not feeling great yet. Two DIFFICULT chapters down, several more to go.

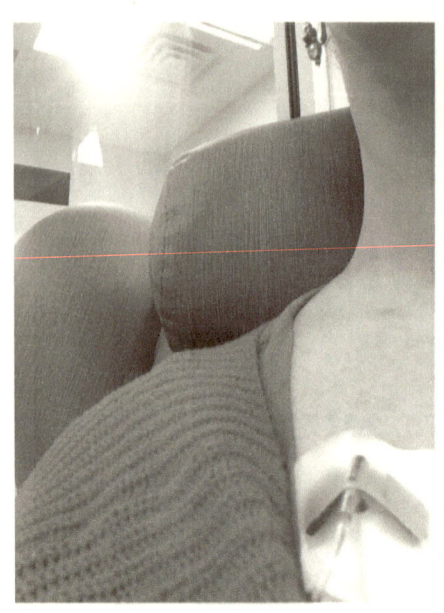
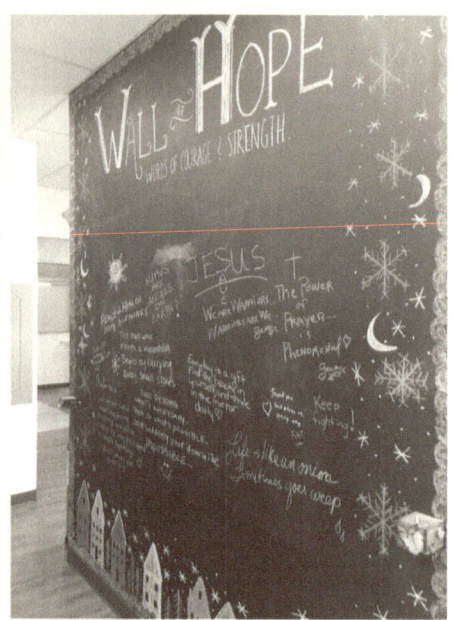

* * *

DECEMBER 31, 2017

Happy New Year!
F.U. Old Year!

T om and I have been saving champagne corks for about 20 years. This one got a double message. Happy New Year 2018! We made it!! Phew!! 😄

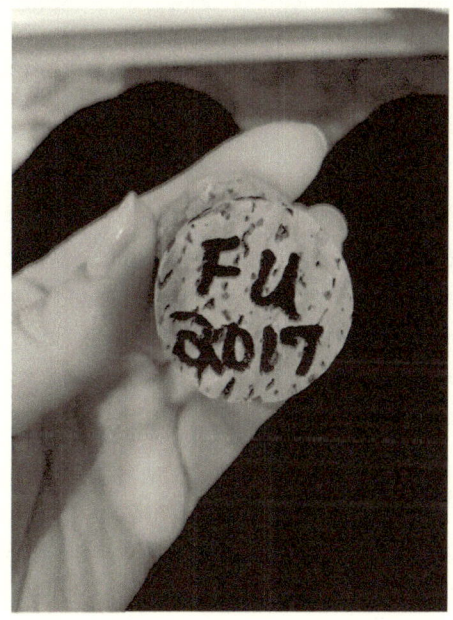

RADIATION

Round 3, Ding! Ding! Ding!

I kissed off 2017 knowing that I had two big, horrible chapters behind me in this journey and THAT'S the truth! Round three began today: radiation. That was after infusion #9 out of 18. Oh, and physical therapy. I had my Wonder Woman socks on the whole day!

Recovery from the mastectomy wasn't the easiest. As you know by now, it was super emotional for me. But I also ended up with something called "axillary cording." It can happen when they take lymph nodes. There is a literal cord, it looks like a tendon but it's not, going from my armpit to my wrist. It felt like my arm was tethered to my side and it was super painful to raise. I have to go to physical therapy for it to be corrected. I don't have full range of motion (yet), but gained a lot of degrees over the weekend, thankfully. Another sucky thing? My bald spot is filling in. In SILVER! It looks like I'm wearing a silver yarmulke.

Oh, and hot flashes are KILLER. Ladies, all the ladies, my condolences if you've had to deal with these internal infernos. On the plus side, I like to think of myself as having "had" cancer. To me, the chemo shrunk it, the mastectomy sent it packing. The radiation is there as an insurance policy. That doesn't mean I'm happy about having to go. Of course, the infusions will continue until next August.

Otherwise, I have turned some small corners. My stamina is coming back a little bit. I do mostly feel like myself from 7:30 AM to 7:30 PM, but I hit a wall at some point in the day. I absolutely have to be careful to conserve my energy right now.

I had my initial radiation consult two weeks ago. Because I couldn't raise my arm over my head (yet) and then leave it there for 20 minutes to do a body cast, we had to hold off starting radiation. But I went today for the casting, tattooing and simulation. Now I know that I will have 32 rounds of daily radiation, Monday through Friday, starting next Thursday. 26 rounds will go to the general area and then 6 rounds will go to the scar itself.

Particularly painful information that also came out of all of this is that reconstruction cannot be considered for three to four years now. It had initially been one to two years, but changed due to the inflammatory nature of this beast.

Say it with me -- THAT SUCKS! (Thank you for indulging me. That is sometimes all I need to hear.) I have tentatively navigated the waters of prosthetics -- they are SO heavy! But another angel approached me and knitted one for me! Any knitters out there that have exhausted their families with scarves and hats? Knitters for Knitted Knockers are knitting FREE ones for mastectomy patients! You pick the cup size, you pick the color, you pick with a nipple or without! Amazing people are out there. I have been astonished by the depth of their generosity.

They said I should be feeling more like myself in six months to a year from now. 😟🔫 I do feel like it's been long enough at this point...But do you know what? I have found myself singing again...dancing in the kitchen again. I went food shopping by myself. I was never so happy to see my eyebrow hairs (it now seems absurd that I waxed them for so many years). I was able to run up the steps to the high school swim meet observation deck this week (I had to pull myself up in November and December, if I could go at all).

It turns out my kids are NOT happy that I know all (most, now) of the words to Bust a Move. I had THOUGHT they would be so proud of me!! But I know they were happy to see me again like they have always previously known me. I was also able to override chemo brain to start AND finish a book. I have even signed up for a continuing education seminar.

The biggest side effect of radiation will be fatigue. After so many, many months of feeling so very bad, the last week or two has given me a glimmer of normalcy again. I'm preparing for the possibility that I might be REALLY tired again, but that's OK, I can do it. Especially with so many blessings. Oh, and three new tattoos. Because I told you in the beginning I was a badass.

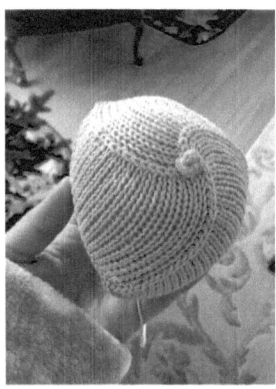
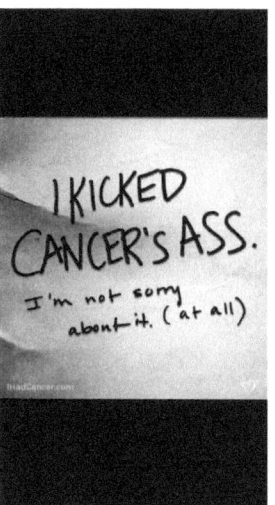

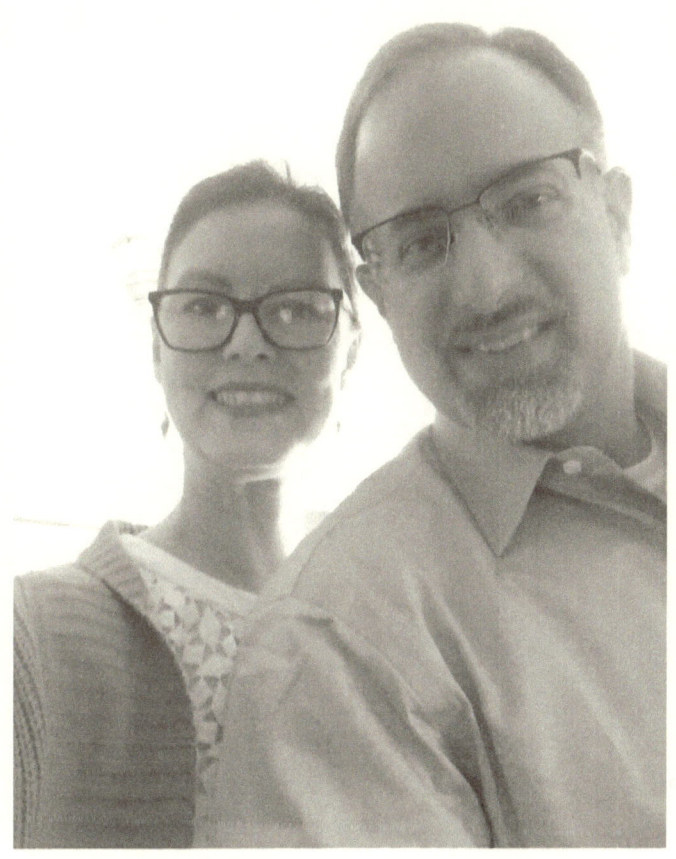

TATTOOS

Lefties Live in their Right Brains (and Right Hearts)

So, what did YOU do today? I got another tattoo, my fourth in a week. Bad ass, remember? But these were due to the radiation treatments I started yesterday and the need for me to be in the perfect position when I'm laser beamed. I guess four tattoos gets me in just the right position. Radiation in relation to the other treatments? Not so bad. Chemotherapy is TERRIBLE. A mastectomy is TERRIBLE.

But radiation is very relatable. How so? Most people by now have had an MRI or a CT scan. It just seems like I'm going into an awfully familiar space, although still in an uncomfortable way. I didn't burst out my leaking tears yesterday or today, like I have in the past.

Afterwards, I teared up a couple of times over the course of the day, simply because it still all sucks. And I wasn't prepared to feel immediate skin burning. According to one of the therapists, that CAN happen if one has "wicked sensitive" skin. Check that box for me. But, after today, two down, thirty to go.

My mom came with me yesterday, Tom came with me today. As we were walking in, Tom muttered, "I hate this fucking place." It's so weird, because I was also thinking the same. The hospital workers are lovely, the treatments are regarded as miraculous. But, on any given day, I'd rather be anywhere else but there.

I'm NOT looking forward to the associated fatigue. Cancer healing is NOT easy for a Type A personality. I go round and round with this. And I'm NOT good at sitting around. Otherwise, I'm trying to (ever the multitasker) meditate while getting the radiation, but the irony is too hard to bear.

A lot of people have commented about my lack of microwave here. I was not afraid of the radiation coming off of it (although it would behoove everybody to look up EMFs and their relation to health). Most people know that I spend a ton of time talking food and actually cooking. What it came down to was this: WHY would I care about the quality of food I buy for my family AND spend the time to buy it, prepare it, if microwaving KILLS all of the micronutrients and enzymes in the food?

I also held off on x-raying my children at the dentist until we get to orthodontic time. So, to lie there GETTING radiated is a RIDICULOUS concept to me, but I will keep my focus on the radiation beams blasting out black, oily, disgusting cancer cells and planting abundant pink, voluptuous flowers that are crazy bold in their bodaciousness. That's the imagery I return to most. I remember reading years ago that green superfoods (spirulina, broccoli sprouts, etc.) and sea vegetables help clear the body of radiation so, "I'd like a green superfood smoothie for one, please!"

You know I've said that writing these posts is extremely cathartic for me. What also helps is asking you all about your experiences with this, if you have them. I hear great stories and they give me massive hope. But I hear heartbreaking stories, too, which would be impossible not to hear when I'm in interviewing mode. I try to learn what I can from these sad stories and regroup.

There have been two patterns that I keep noticing. It started with a conversation in my kitchen. A friend's mom had unilateral breast cancer, left side. My friend told me that every time her mom had to go to the hospital, the kids were told that their mom was getting her tonsils out. And then, another friend, I spoke to at the Community Center recently: her mom had unilateral breast cancer, left side. Every time HER mom went to the hospital, my friend thought she was having a baby.

The pattern became easy to spot: left side, hidden emotions. I actually made a list of how many of my friends told me that their mom had breast cancer. I thought I would research this leftsidedness -- but a quick Google search showed me that "many studies have shown that unilateral breast cancer is more frequent in the left breast than in the right." Where our hearts are. I had NO idea.

Thank God I can emote about this. Thank God my kids can know EXACTLY what is going on, age appropriately. Thank God I don't have to hide, because thinking about your moms and how society worked in such a way that these overworked and underappreciated moms had to have their hearts breaking privately, I've thought about them so, so much. And I've thought about you, too, and how you were just kids like mine. I can emote about this thanks to your moms and you.

Maybe they would think that I'm a gigantic baby for doing this in such a public and vocal way, but I've been thanked more than once by their daughters for being honest with my kids about this and it has become yet another blessing that I am thankful for. I came across a post on Facebook recently by Cancer Warrioress and, while not exactly science, it makes the most sense to me. She wrote it in a post called "Healing Heartbreak" on 1/6 of this year.

"I felt how my body ingeniously grew this tumor over my heart

as the agony was too much to bear. I had to protect myself and thus, the cancer within me took root. When Deb was diagnosed and I slowly watched my beloved friend be ravaged by cancer, the tumor grew larger. When Deb died and I bid farewell to my twin soul sister, the grief threatened once again to tear me apart. I know the grief, loss and cancer were all one. The heart bleeds tears of sadness for the departed.

It feels healthy to cry these tears remembering how deeply I loved. It feels healing to let the layer of armor melt away and remember the beauty that was shared. Life goes on and there is still so much to be thankful for.

I share this with you as we all carry wounds within us. I believe the key to true healing is to allow our hearts to speak the pain they hold. Share your grief. Speak your sorrow. If not now, then when?

And in the precious memories of times long gone, laughter shared, vows made, friends whom have passed, relationships released, there is beauty, love and a recognition that we have lived our lives the best we could, shattered hearts and all. In our vulnerability there is truth and healing.

Thank you for witnessing my vulnerability."

I couldn't have said it better if I tried for a million years. It's really something that these unilateral breast cancers seem to show up around the time of major hormonal shifts, whether it's the onset of menses, childbearing, perimenopause, menopause, etc. It's what defines us as women, but don't hold the stress in, please, oh, pretty please. Don't hold in your stress.

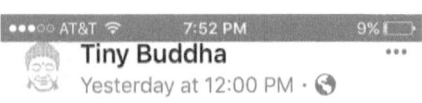

●●●○○ AT&T 🛜　　7:52 PM　　9% 🔋

Tiny Buddha
Yesterday at 12:00 PM · 🌐

"It will get better. There is a meaning to what you're going through. You will feel like living again. If you can't do anything else but breathe, do just that; you don't have to do anything else. Don't fight it. Let it be. It is as it should be and it's okay. Just be. Don't judge. Let go. Look at what's beautiful. Listen to what gives you peace. Eat what tastes good. Do what feels nice. Even if it feels pointless right now, it's good for your soul. Ask for help. Let other people help you. Let other people take care of you. Cry. Scream. Wail. Laugh. Sleep. Close your eyes. Do whatever you need to do. Let it out. And embrace. It will get

●●●○○ AT&T 🛜　　7:52 PM　　9% 🔋

your soul. Ask for help. Let other people help you. Let other people take care of you. Cry. Scream. Wail. Laugh. Sleep. Close your eyes. Do whatever you need to do. Let it out. And embrace. It will get better. I promise." ~Helena Önneby

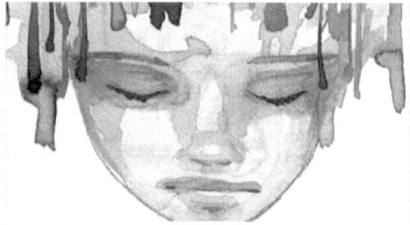

A First Aid Kit for When Life Falls Apart - Tiny Buddha
tinybuddha.com

👍❤️😮 2.4K　　　　133 Comments

👍 Like　💬 Comment　↪ Share

RADIATION CONTINUES

February 19, 2018

56%

As of today, I am 18 daily radiations down, with 14 to go. That makes me exactly 56 percent done with radiation.

As of my last infusion, I am 10 Herceptin infusions down, 8 to go. That makes me exactly 56 percent done with infusions.

Both are 56 percent done. TODAY?? That was a little shocking to me. What are the chances? But I don't really have much to say about radiation. I was GOING to post at the halfway point, 16 down, 16 to go, on Thursday. That felt momentous, except it was the day after the Florida school shooting, so my heart wasn't into spewing about any annoyances of radiation. I feel heartsick about what happened in Florida and the families directly involved.

But I've heard from a lot of you now, reaching out to see how I'm doing, so I figured that I would bring everybody up to date. Thank you for reaching out, my loves. Here's my current deal.

I am not proud of this, but it turns out that I'm a cutthroat

radiationer. Radiationist? Radiationizer? Radiationalist? Radi-
ationee? As in -- by the time the elderly couple parking next to
me makes it into the radiation waiting room, in their hospital
gowns, I am already running out of the radiation machine room.
I am hopping over slow people, running around the side of the
people who have stopped to talk to people they recognize. I
would probably appear unfriendly there. I don't want to stop
and talk. I'm not there to make friends. For God's sake, I don't
want to run into anyone I know there. I almost always (politely)
turn down offers from friends to take me. I appreciate your
offers, it is SO sweet of you, from the bottom of my heart, truly.

But, if I can get in to the hospital and back out in record time (I
constantly play beat the clock), later in the day I can almost forget that I've been there. Tom took me today -- holy moly was I
fast. He pulled up, I jumped out of the car. By the time he parked
and he sat down in the waiting room, I was already running out,
done for today. Get me the fuck out of here. That's how I feel,
each and every day. It's daily.

So, I can forget about it until my radiated area starts tingling
later in the day. But, it's not even that bad. I was afraid it would
be when I started stinging and burning the very first day. Turns
out that they forgot I was allergic to adhesive. Now that I have
THAT situated, it has only been very light tingling and stinging
so far. I am told to moisturize, moisturize, moisturize. That's
one side effect of radiation.

So far, so good, with 14 more to go. And, oddly enough, there is
a Wonder Woman aloe bottle in the radiation dressing room's
bathroom. I give her a quick nod and a "how the hell are ya?," say
a silent thank you for the strength she inspires in me. Her bottle
has been empty for a while now, but I don't think any patients or
staff can give her the heave ho. I know I can't.

It's the fatigue that's starting to gain on me. While I MAY have
a night where I stay up until 10:30 or 11:00, it almost always comes with nights of being asleep on the couch by 7:30

or 8:00. TOTALLY BORING to my former Party Girl ways. Of all the things I miss from my life B.C., it's my former stamina that I miss most. But, truth be told, I can look back and realize that I was starting to lose ground in the year before I was diagnosed. Everything felt like it was getting harder and harder. I just thought that it was middle age catching up on me, I never thought it was what it turned out to be. So fatigue is my second radiation symptom.

And now for my third symptom. The one that grew in me because of my Shannonism and now is taking up my hours when I'm not radiating or sleeping. Organizing. Because I felt like I was losing ground before the diagnosis and then (as someone who NEEDS my ducks in a row) had my ducks tossed warp-speed into the universe, ducks that were procreating like bunnies, so there were FAMILIES of my ducks that I didn't recognize but still needed to gather.

There is a slight terror in the back of my head. While I am planning to live to 100, while I do believe I will pull through this, while I am not focusing on the negative, there is that WHAT IF factor. WHAT IF. Don't tell me not to go there. I dare you not to if you were in my shoes. I don't dwell on it, but it's always there. Don't tell me that there were never any guarantees about my life expectancy. While true, once you receive a diagnosis of cancer, it is ALWAYS in the back of your head. Don't think you know how you'd be upon hearing similar news. I'm not following any script of how I thought I'd be.

On dark days I think, "What if we had to sell the house? What if Tom and the kids had to figure out my systems that I had put into place along the way of child-rearing? What if my plans for my kids didn't come to fruition?" Oh, I know they'd be okay. They're good kids. But I don't want them wondering about anything.

For example, what was I PLANNING on doing with those weird piles of t-shirts stored away in the basement? For your information, they are the kids' former FAVORITE t-shirts of all their teams, hobbies, etc., to be made into quilts for them for their high school graduations.

Or, that strange pile of recipes in a box? Family favorites to pass down to them. That one box of Christmas decorations that never comes out? Decorations that their grandmother made, that I'd like to pass down to them when they have their first homes.

So, what IF?? Well, I am partially wanting to get jump started on the legacy I was going to leave them someday. But it's probably more like I have felt like I've had NO control for a while now, so I'm trying to control the shit out of that closet. And that closet. And that closet. And get stuff to people that is not getting used here.

I have never been a consumer. You would be astounded on how little I spend on "stuff." But I don't want anything here that doesn't have a purpose. I have jumped on that Lent bandwagon of getting rid of 40 bags in 40 days. I also gave up gluten. So far, so good. I'm experimenting on getting rid of inflammatory things.

I'm hoping that the WHAT IF part, that sometimes makes me lose my breath, that sometimes makes me feel like I have anxiety for literally the first time in my life, that I try to mitigate through prayer and meditation, WHAT IF I just finally have my house organized? But what if I die young? What if I beat this? What if I am destined to do something in my life that I didn't see coming? That I never would have known without having met this cancer first? But WHAT IF I could just find my favorite sweater that I've been missing for a while?

That would make me happy today. Just to solve some little mysteries that have been bugging me. And, at the very least, get me away from the specter of a cancer diagnosis for a little while. After all, you can't take it with you and I don't really want Tom and the kids to wonder what I wanted to do with any of it.

I CAN say this -- the china? The silver? The crystal I registered for when we got married? It came out on Wednesday night. Tom, the kids and I had a formal dinner in the dining room on Valentine's Day. They won't have to wonder what to do with it. You USE it. It doesn't collect dust in the cabinets. And, by the way, the kids acted with more manners in the dining room. Who knew?

The next phase of my care brings along a medication that is dastardly. The oncologist said he hardly ever prescribes it because he knows how hard the last 8 months have been and then to throw a drug at me that has terrible symptoms he knows is emotionally hard. He said I could SAFELY wait to start it for 2-1/2 years. I would take it for a year, but the first month would be the most terrible.

There is a reason I had my kids close together. I knew that if I saw the light at the end of the tunnel, I might not go back to having babies. I feel the same way about this: just get it over with. That was a NOT FUN conversation. More on that when I start living the fourth installment of cancer care.

In the meantime, I'm still stuck on the third phase, that interlude chapter that you know, if YOU were the writer of that book, you wouldn't have included and the book would have felt exactly the same. For me, it is all the agricultural conversations in Anna Karenina. That's this chapter of mine. Boring, still necessary to the author for some reason but I find myself just RACING through it. At least 56 percent of the day, I'm racing through it because I'm exhausted through the rest of it.

Oh, I know that we were never in control. Prayers help me get back on that horse. I refer to the prayer Footprints ALL of the time. In the meantime, someone I know that's very wise asked me in the beginning of this ridiculousness if there were something I've always wanted to do, but never had the time. She meant well -- she thought I would have extra time on my hands right now. I don't, but she asked me if there was a language I've always wanted to learn? A college course I wanted to do online? A new hobby? Besides just my regular stuff I have to do, anti-cancering takes up A LOT of time but it did get me thinking.

What would I want to put more time into if I had the time? I can tell you one thing right now. Gun control. Not to get political. I am, while not newly on board, I am newly PASSIONATELY on board. What would you put time into if you had the time? I'm curious. I'd love to know. Because I'm 56 percent done with some of this fucking shit. Pardon my French. It's F-word day.

Credit for excerpt of poem below - Jenn Brenner.

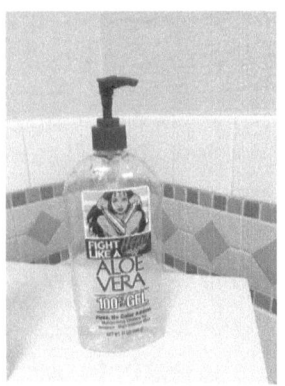
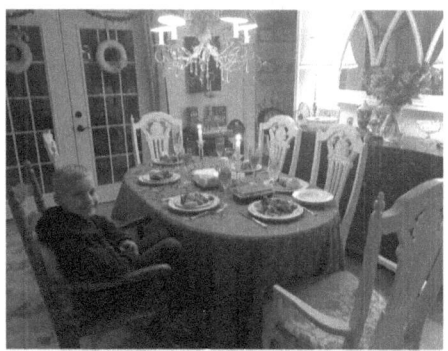

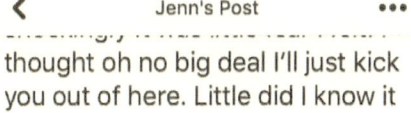

<   Jenn's Post   •••

thought oh no big deal I'll just kick
you out of here. Little did I know it
would take a lot more than that
dear.

You like to make your presence
known by causing so much pain.
Feelings of uncertainty and tears
that fall like rain.
I can honestly say I never thought
why did we have to meet. It may
sound insane but I felt relieved
that you chose me. I wouldn't want
it to be any of the women I love
you see.

I could sit here and bash you until
no end. But this is about a thank

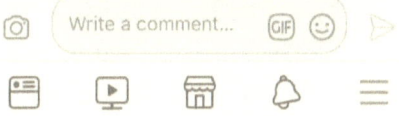

THE MOUNTAIN LION

February 28, 2018

This is exactly how I've been feeling this week. Don't ask me about it, please. I might burst out crying. I was not sure who the original author was initially, but silently thanked that bad-ass chick anyway. A quick Google search brought me to Caitlin Feeley, and a blog called Dread Pirate Khan. Seven more radiations to go, and I'm not feeling so terrific. I saw it on Facebook one day, it's been reposted millions of times. The best I could initially gather was "Some Hedgehog" wrote it on a Blog post but I could not verify that. But it speaks TO me. It speaks FOR me. And I'm quite sure it does the same for other survivors.

> *"What's it like to go through cancer treatment? It's something like this: one day, you're minding your own business, you open the fridge to get some breakfast, and OH MY GOD THERE'S A MOUNTAIN LION IN YOUR FRIDGE.*

Wait, what? How? Why is there a mountain lion in your fridge? NO TIME TO EXPLAIN. RUN! THE MOUNTAIN LION WILL KILL YOU! UNLESS YOU FIND SOMETHING EVEN MORE FEROCIOUS TO KILL IT FIRST!

So you take off running, and the mountain lion is right behind you. You know the only thing that can kill a mountain lion is a bear, and the only bear is on top of the mountain, so you better find that bear. You start running up the mountain in hopes of finding the bear. Your friends desperately want to help, but they are powerless against mountain lions, as mountain lions are godless killing machines. But they really want to help, so they're cheering you on and bringing you paper cups of water and orange slices as you run up the mountain and yelling at the mountain lion - "GET LOST, MOUNTAIN LION, NO ONE LIKES YOU" - and you really appreciate the support, but the mountain lion is still coming.

Also, for some reason, there's someone in the crowd who's yelling "that's not really a mountain lion, it's a puma" and another person yelling "I read that mountain lions are allergic to kale, have you tried rubbing kale on it?"

As you're running up the mountain, you see other people fleeing their own mountain lions. Some of the mountain lions seem comparatively wimpy - they're half grown and only have three legs or whatever, and you think to yourself - why couldn't I have gotten one of those mountain lions? But then you look over at the people who are fleeing mountain lions the size of a monster truck with huge prehistoric saber fangs, and you feel like an asshole for even thinking that -- and besides, who in their right mind would want to fight a mountain lion, even a three-legged one?

Finally, the person closest to you, whose job it is to take care of you -- maybe a parent or sibling or best friend or, in my case, my husband -- comes barging out of the woods and jumps on the mountain lion, whaling on it and screaming "GODDAM-MIT MOUNTAIN LION, STOP TRYING TO EAT MY WIFE," and the mountain lion punches your husband right in the face. Now your husband (or whatever) is rolling around on the ground clutching his nose, and he's bought you some time, but you still need to get to the top of the mountain.

Eventually you reach the top, finally, and the bear is there. Waiting. For both of you. You rush right up to the bear, and the bear rushes the mountain lion, but the bear has to go through you to get to the mountain lion, and in doing so, the bear TOTALLY KICKS YOUR ASS, but not before it also punches your husband in the face. And your husband is now stagger-ing around with a black eye and bloody nose, and saying "can I get some help, I've been punched in the face by two apex predators and I think my nose is broken," and all you can say is "I'M KIND OF BUSY IN CASE YOU HADN'T NOTICED I'M FIGHTING A MOUNTAIN LION."

Then, IF YOU ARE LUCKY, the bear leaps on the mountain lion and they are locked in epic battle until finally the two of them roll off a cliff edge together, and the mountain lion is dead.

Maybe. You're not sure - it fell off the cliff, but mountain lions are crafty. It could come back at any moment.

And all your friends come running up to you and say "that was amazing! You're so brave, we're so proud of you! You didn't die! That must be a huge relief!"

Meanwhile, you blew out both your knees, you're having an asthma attack, you twisted your ankle, and also you have been mauled by a bear. And everyone says "boy, you must be excited to walk down the mountain!" And all you can think as you stagger to your feet is, "Fuck this mountain, I never wanted to climb it in the first place."

LAST OF THE BIG 3 FINALE

March 9, 2018

Praying

N umber three of the "big three" done today. Radiation is done! I ended up with 31 visits, and it was easily the most benign of the big treatments thus far. My skin doesn't feel great, but it never broke open or blistered. It really just looks like a moderate sunburn. Besides the burning and itching, the biggest symptom has been fatigue. Building back my stamina is my first order of business. I'll be happy not to make that daily trip to the hospital that I did for approximately six weeks. No FOMO there for me!

My husband and my sister both nominated me for a "Diva for a Day" opportunity and I received word that they chose me. So I'm looking forward to decompressing at a day spa soon, thanks to the donations given to that nonprofit looking out for women in their shocking diagnosis year.

Speaking of the word shocking: can you believe, eight months into this, I am STILL in shock? I had a breakdown of sorts recently. It was like I had gotten the diagnosis all over again, fresh and new. The same anxiety threw itself into the mix, the exact same emotional reactions. Thankfully, Tom and the boys were all camping and special friends of mine and Claire's threw a ton of TLC all over us girls. It turns out that this is a very real, natural reaction. From the moment I walked out of that 7/7/17 mammogram, I jumped onto a very fast-moving local train. It often felt like it was going to jump the rails and I was hanging on for dear life. But there was never any question of what stop was next.

The stations were...

Four Biopsies!

Labwork!

Genetic counselor!

More lab work!

Breast MRI

Second look Ultrasound!

2 more biopsies!

Follow-up mammogram!

Meet with surgeon!

Meet with oncologist!

CTs Chest, Abdomen, Pelvis!

Whole Body Scan!

Echocardiogram!

MUGA Scan!

Port Insertion!

Chemo and Infusion #1!

Chemo and Infusion #2!

Wig appointments!

Chemo and Infusion #3!

Chemo and Infusion #4!

Chemo and Infusion #5!

Chemo and Infusion #6!

Premastectomy class!

Echocardiogram #2!

Presurgical consult!

Mammogram and Ultrasound!

Medical clearance appointment!

Infusion #7!

Left simple mastectomy!

Infusion #8!

Radiation consult!

Physical Therapies #1-8!

Infusion #9!

Radiations #1-8...

Infusion #10!

Radiations #9-20!

Echocardiogram #3!

Radiations #21-23!

Infusion #11!

Radiations #24-31!

There were also stops at Reiki, Jin Shin Jyutsu, Healing Touch, massage therapists, social workers, cups of tea over tears, homemade meals, I know they were made with love. That's the way they tasted. Store gift cards, a $20 bill tucked in a card, pink bracelets and blue t-shirts. More pink bracelets. That incredible Breast Cancer walk, I NEVER, EVER would've expected all of those magnificent people on my team. Thanks for walking at my side. There was even a beautiful evening out -- shoutout to Minette's Angels.

A local cleaning company (MaidPro) came in and cleaned our house for the holidays. The owner devotes time from her cleaning business to taking care of cancer patients pro bono. A beautiful pink wig that I will never part with.

And just when I began to wonder how in the world I would ever pull off a Christmas for four kids with a major surgery twelve days before Christmas, in arrived Santa's sleigh, in the form of two departments from the hospital that adopted our family for the holidays. I almost said no. My normal type A personality told me I could pull it off on top of everything else. But this email arrived in my inbox: "I know it is not easy for people to accept help. I would encourage you to do it. Remember, we all need help/offer help at points in time. My guess is, you've helped many, many people and now you get to receive. The world couldn't function if we didn't have both giver and receiver." The thanks goes to Kristy Case, a beautiful social worker from the hospital.

Insert the ugly cry and a humble yes, please, we would be so grateful. The aforementioned recent anxiety? Because after so long of knowing (kind of) what to expect next, now it feels like the guardrails are off.

As for where I left off in my 7/25/17 post, "In the meantime, that inner badass I have? She's almost back. I'm still conjuring her up. I know she'll be here again in just a minute. 💚💚 I'm waiting for her here at the train station now."

And now, back to today:

I just came screeching into that train station. I'm taking a look around, probably kissing the ground. It's been a wild ride -- a white knuckler. But I was holding on -- oh, so very tight. There was no alternative. There's A LOT of sights to see here and a chance to catch my breath, to contemplate the life lessons I am supposed to be gleaning from this. I'll be putting a call into Livestrong, the program at some local Ys to build cancer patients back up to their fighting level. I am REALLY tired.

But I'm gathering up some of the other badass women I've met in my journey. The two survivors that tucked me up under their own Wonder Women capes. Other wonderful women who were bold enough to tell me their stories while keeping their stories on the private side. Their secrets are safe with me. And the FIVE NEWLY diagnosed women, only since my July diagnosis, that I already knew socially. Some are quietly noble and some publicly proud, all wearing their own version of Wonder Women socks for bravery, the visual reminder to be brave for ourselves and our families when courage is hard to summon up organically.

On the way home from the hospital today, I heard that new song by Kesha, Pray. I know it's about a predator. Thank God she came out on the other side of her horror show stronger than ever and giving many hope. To me, that song loosely translates to the predator of cancer and all of those fighting. This song had me in a parking spot, head on the wheel, crying a few weeks ago. For about two minutes. And then I sort of looked around and thought, "Okay! That's out! Done now!"

You know I have to interject some Foo Fighters, too. Because also in my feed today, footage of All My Life from their most recent concert. Done, done and I'm on to the next one. Another example of art imitating life. Two more songs in my Beast Mode playlist.

Next station stops this year: Infusions #12 through 18. Not much to see at those stops. Keep moving, keep moving, heading out of the busy city and into the suburbs. More space between stops now and more room to move around, spread out on that train, take a breath, take in the beautiful landscape. Just don't fall asleep, forget where you're going and wind up at the end of the line. But, I'm on a TRAIN CAR WITH BADASSES!!! My family, which goes without saying, and, oh my goodness, survivor/thriver ladies -- you have all carried me and I'm getting ready to carry you, if you need me!

Off to unpack that radiation bag. I won't be needing THAT one anymore! So nice to lighten my load. What a SPECIAL St. Patrick's Day week to celebrate.

PRAYING, by Kesha

Well, you almost had me fooled

Told me that I was nothing without you

Oh, but after everything you've done

I can thank you for how strong I have become

'Cause you brought the flames and you put me through hell

I had to learn how to fight for myself

And we both know all the truth I could tell

I'll just say this is "I wish you farewell"

I hope you're somewhere prayin', prayin'

I hope your soul is changin', changin'

I hope you find your peace

Falling on your knees, prayin'

I'm proud of who I am

No more monsters, I can breathe again

And you said that I was done

Well, you were wrong and now the best is yet to come

'Cause I can make it on my own, oh

And I don't need you, I found a strength I've never known

I'll bring thunder, I'll bring rain, oh

When I'm finished, they won't even know your name

You brought the flames and you put me through hell

I had to learn how to fight for myself

And we both know all the truth I could tell

I'll just say this is "I wish you farewell"

I hope you're somewhere prayin', prayin'

I hope your soul is changin', changin'

I hope you find your peace

Falling on your knees, prayin'

Ah sometimes, I pray for you at night, oh

Someday, maybe you'll see the light

Whoa oh oh oh, some say, in life, you're gonna get what you give

But some things only God can forgive

Yeah! (I hope you're somewhere prayin', prayin')

I hope your soul is changin', changin'

I hope you find your peace

Falling on your knees, prayin'

ESTROGEN (FOO)FIGHTER

Holy Shit

This chapter might be more boring than the others. It's kind of a picking up the pieces chapter -- a HOLY SHIT chapter, what the HELL happened to me chapter. It lacks the horror of Chapters 1 (diagnosis and chemo) and 2 (mastectomy), the drudgery of Chapter 3 (radiation). There is an element of trying to figure out how to start over with this new normal, but thankfully, there is SOME breathing room. This is the "lots of happy pills for you" chapter (for you Monty Python fans). It's the Tamoxifen chapter and oh, here's your prescription, it's for a DECADE.

Does everybody remember my holistic career? This doesn't jibe for me at all. Here's what I am told to expect with Tamoxifen: mega hot flashes, lots of joint pain and about a 30 pound weight gain. Nice, right? I had a Breast Cancer Index test done this week. It gives me a 15 percent chance of reoccurrence five to ten years after diagnosis. It was hard for me not to hear 85 percent non-reoccurrence, but my oncologist said that the numbers usually seen are 6-9 percent. So, Tamoxifen it is. Again, I know I'm not a number, but UGH.

I'm sitting at my infusion (#14 out of 18) right now -- the tri-weekly "miracle" infusion of Herceptin, due to my Her-2 protein indication that we always knew would continue for a full calendar year. There are three things you should know here:

1) You avid wordsmiths already know that triweekly means both occurring every three weeks AND occurring three times per week. For the record, it's every three weeks. There are practically no symptoms from these infusions. But I am still in the chemo chair and they would win me over better if they put me in a pedicure chair for this. I tend to get tired and headachy later in the week after the infusion but that's about it. Fourteen down, four to go.

2) There is actually a movie out there with Harry Connick, Jr. detailing the discovery of Herceptin. The drug almost didn't see the light of day. There was a lot of dumb luck to get this miracle drug to the masses. I have not seen it but that's how monumental this drug is thought to be, that a whole movie was made in it's honor. It changed the prognoses of triple positive women like crazy -- from pretty grim to much less so.

3) The Herceptin discovery actually came from money donated to the American Cancer Society. This makes me feel all the better about doing the Breast Cancer Awareness Making Strides walk in October. I will be there again.

And now, we come to the topic of Estrogen. Take THAT, Estrogen. Back OFF, Estrogen! Don't come around these parts NO MO', Estrogen! You might remember that my previous cancer diagnosis ate Estrogen like candy. Estrogen fed the flames of this cancer. You know what Estrogen does -- it makes girls look like they are blooming flowers. Their skin looks like a perfectly ripe fruit. It eventually makes babies and feeds them, too. Estrogen is supposed to be good for us! We have run into trouble here in the industrial world. Because NOW we have Estrogen mimickers. Tons and tons and tons. But wait -- more tons. Chemicals that have gone into our bodies and PRETEND to be Estrogen.

I'm starting to regret capitalizing the word Estrogen. Autocorrect keeps making me. I am now going to override autocorrect, because estrogen has already tried to take over my life. Nothing doing, estrogen. Take THAT, asshole. Obvious estrogen mimickers are pesticides. Your grass looks lush, but I wouldn't want my kids to play near your house. But, shoot, one rainstorm and they are playing in it, inadvertently. It also renews my commitment to buying organic food. I shudder when I walk my dog and watch your children playing on your grass where pesticide flags say no children or animals. Dandelions were THAT preposterous to you? Weeds? Com on now. Do better for your children.

There are other things that mimic estrogen-- your regular beauty products, new car smell, anything with synthetic fragrance. I have known this and have lectured about these chemicals for years. But I was unprepared for this one -- the levels of BPA are very high in cash register receipts, and the more you handle receipts, the more BPA is in your system. Cashiers have higher concentrations of it in their bloodstream. So I have to take this drug that blocks the effects of estrogen while trying to avoid estrogen anyway.

It's a real somebody done somebody wrong song, with me and my messy, messy attempt to divorce from estrogen. Soy and it's derivatives really mess these things up for my (and probably your) health, too. Especially genetically modified. For a real kick, you should try to find a salad dressing without soy in it. You'll find them, but good luck with that!

Yes, Morris Plains residents, I have a "Say NO to Mane" sign on my front lawn. Synthetic fragrance is one of the major causes of allergies and estrogen assault. I have avoided it for years, so many that I can't even go down the laundry aisle in a food store

-- those smells are sickening to me! Thank you to those who are leading this crusade of blocking a CHEMICAL company in our 2-3 square mile town. Doesn't the concept look ridiculous on paper?? It SOUNDS like the MOST ABSURD thing to me. Anyway, I know this much is true: every single time I present to a practitioner and we talk about my having no risk factors and no genetic component for breast cancer, the next statement is, "it must be environmental."

I remember hearing a talk once about how EVERY single dollar you spend is a political decision. We have talked a lot about this in our house.

"Mommy? Why don't you buy {insert bad company product here}?"

"Well, my love, that company doesn't care about our health/ environment/lives. And I'm not going to make that company richer if they don't."

That didn't always do it for them and I found myself resorting to, "I must love you more than the other people who buy that product love themselves." Listen -- no offense, people might not know yet. But once you know, you can't UNKNOW. And you don't have to tell me that you saw my kids at QuickChek buying Gatorade the other day. I know all about it.

Come to think of it, I am also suspicious of companies that spell their names phonetically. They think we are STUPID, people!! Demand that what comes into your house be from companies who care. We wouldn't "need" fragrance chemical manufacturing companies in our towns if we didn't "need" them in our homes, if we stopped buying fragrances or demanded safety. It is SO interesting to check out what chemicals are banned in socialist countries -- when they have to pay for the healthcare, the unhealthy things come out of the system.

By the way, my infusions are much shorter than the chemo treatments. I have sat in this chair 14 times now. Part of what doesn't make it easy is to see no one even close to my age sitting in here. But I think it just got worse today. A pregnant lady just walked in and got hooked up to her chemo IV. God's honest truth. Her estrogen got her, too. It was supposed to be helping her.

In other news, I cut my hair short. Really short. I had no choice. Tom and my sister nominated me for a "Diva for a Day" for breast cancer patients. It came with a mini facial, massage, manicure, pedicure and make-up application. And a blowout. But there was nothing to blow out. My former bald spot had an inch and a half of hair on top and then I had these Frankenstein pieces surrounding my head. In reality, I had nothing to blow out, so off it went. I also had three hairdressers standing around me with their waving fingers asking, "WHY?? WHY??" Was I trying to keep this look?? They were exasperated. I was trying to explain that it was not the look I was going for. I did not equate what I was looking like with BEAUTY, but the remnants of a life from what I remembered.

And I had met the primary goal. To save my kids from being reminded every second of every day that we were in a scary place this past year. The hairdresser had her job cut out for her. There were pictures posted, but I had just spent the entire time in the chair crying. It represents another thing I lost this year. There are scars, a port, places where there were holes. She asked me if I had naturally curly hair and it SEEMED like such a good idea to pull out a picture that was taken RIGHT before I was diagnosed last summer. BAD IDEA.

It was a picture of me from the first time I ever spent a little money on my hair. I had added highlights. What a waste of money. I only got to enjoy them for a couple of weeks. She also told me that I should start dressing sexy. A little bit of a conundrum since alot of my closet is LL BEAN and Lands' End. Max said to me, "Mommy. I love it. It looks like mine now." But, two weeks later I still don't identify with this 8-year-old boy haircut of mine. So be it. He's happy I look like him for once because I've been asked if I was his nanny with my brown hair and green eyes, next to his blonde hair and blue eyes. Today, we look alike in his eyes. Except for the extra make-up and the BIG ASS earrings I keep reaching for since my hair has been chopped.

I am at a standstill when it comes to the next thing on my list of things to do -- to find a prosthetic bathing suit. Uh-oh, I'm supposed to be dressing sexy, right? Because of my haircut? We took the kids to an overnight at Kalahari right after Thanksgiving (and the completion of chemotherapy) and before my surgery. It was the last time my left breast was seen in public. It was also the last time I would be able to wear my favorite bathing suit. I'm going to miss that one. I have not yet been able to go through my underwear drawer and sort out the upper undergarments that no longer make sense. In due time, I guess.

In terms of work, I had April 15th as the date in my head for going back but I am still dealing with an arm that doesn't function as it should due to the lymph nodes and musculature taken. If I had a desk job? I could probably sit there. But I don't. I also don't have my stamina back at all. I had the good fortune to attend a ball on Thursday night. Thank you to Minette's Angels!! So fun. I danced. I felt like my old self again. But I had nothing to give the next day.

I rallied Saturday and got my Cub Scout troop to a full day at camp. Also so fun. Sunday? Dragging again. SUPER FRUSTRATING, I am used to operating at a fast pace. At the ball, I talked to a 20 year breast cancer survivor about this kind of stuff. She said, in no uncertain terms, "Respect the healing. Respect what your body had to do this year and what it still has to do to get over what it had to do."

So, while I am respecting my body and it's journey, I will keep trying and AS SOON as the Girl Scout cookies are out of my house for the year, you have NO IDEA the kind of respecting I'm going to be doing. The Girl Scout cookies are still just making it a little bit hard right now. But, thank God I wasn't the cookie mom this year. That would have made all of this respecting REALLY hard.

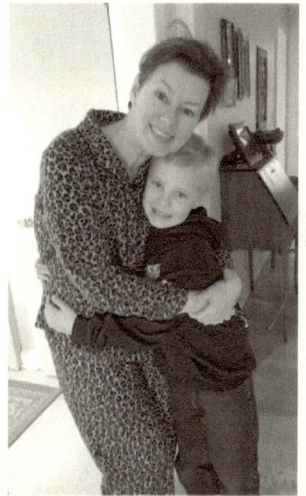

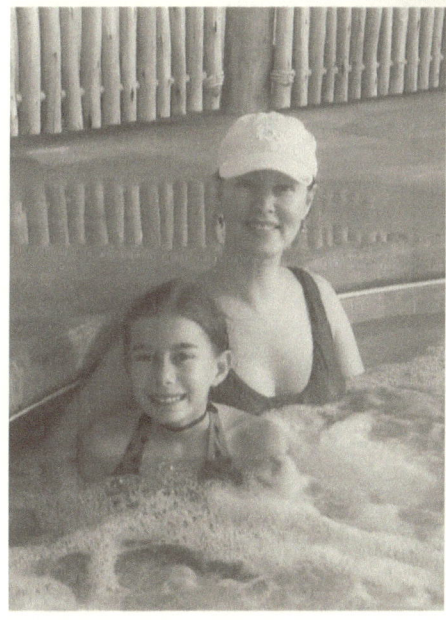

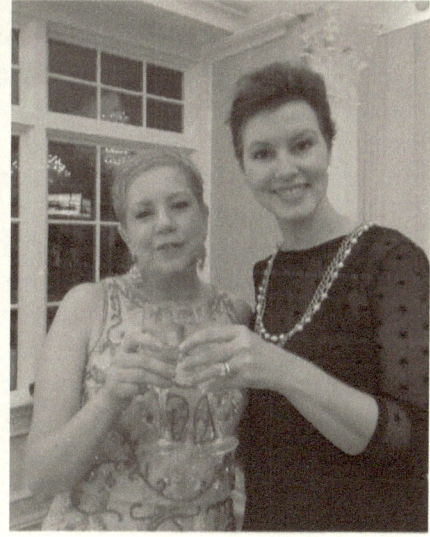

#MOMBOSS IN THE MORNING

June 5, 2018

The best thing thing about this day was heading out to a fancy morning with my breast cancer "mentor" and friend, Judy. I always try step it up a little notch when I head out with her. She's glamorous. We were served mimosas (we survivors love to celebrate with a little champagne day drinking once in a while) and beautiful little breakfast foods, artistically curated for a morning of luxury for harried and hassled moms. I was excited when I got there. We were OUT on the town. Judy had taken me under her wing as a survivor who was almost exactly one year ahead of me on the breast cancer path. Mutual friends told us each that we would have to meet each other to help each other on a journey in a way that only someone else on the same journey can help. We became fast friends and, over time, the friendship began to take on a Thelma and Louise quality. On this particular morning, she had received an invitation to a #MOMBOSS panel of women who were going to share their secrets of success. I was excited to be out on this spring morning, after a year of doctor's appointments and therapies.

Ever the notetaker, I thought I would head home with a bevy of ideas for figuring out the hot mess I was in, thanks to the cancer diagnosis eleven months prior. I was going to reinvent myself! But I guess I wasn't ready yet. It was hard to distance myself from a career that I had long identified with. It was also hard to start from scratch. I wasn't able to work yet. My long term disability plan that I had always been so proud of owning only amounted to $75 a day. Medical bills were starting to arrive by the dozen, followed closely by lawyer's letters threatening suits. I even wrote a lawyer back once. I said something like, "Every time you send a bill threatening a lawsuit, I still have to decide whether I'm going to feed my kids, pay my mortgage or pay your bill. Guess who is going to win, every single time." He still sends me letters and I still pay all of my medical bills $10 a month.

It was instantly clear that these "mom bosses" had incredible access to help, whether it be cleaning ladies, nannies or landscapers. Or even the means to be able to get away from it all with their significant others once in a while. All I wanted back was my "too busy to do my hair" ponytail that in and of itself is a hairstyle in the suburbs. I wanted to JUST GO TO WORK, MAKE A PAYCHECK and worry about what I was going to put in the crockpot for dinner. I said this a lot during my first year -- that I felt like I had been robbed and ransacked. I had NEVER complained about my life. I was happy to wake up to it every single day. I loved the problem solving of it all. And now hard choices needed to be made. We had to consider moving, but couldn't face the prospect of not only the physical burden it would be when I was not up to it, but also now taking the kids' comfort zone away on top of all of the fear and stress of their mom's diagnosis and treatment. There was just no way this could happen.

I sat there wondering about these women's houses and lives and I thought back to mine. I just wanted to go home and organize some closets. It wasn't a jealousy thing with these ladies, just an obvious feeling of living in different worlds and wanting to be back in mine. Maybe I was a little naive before diagnosis, but I had worked HARD and now I had nothing to show for it. My mother had always raised us with the idea that you'll never get more if you're not thankful for what you have. But I had been thankful and now I had so much less.

I tried to remember to be thankful every minute of every day and usually I could turn things around, but cancer is about loss.

Loss of innocence, loss of freedom, loss of body parts, loss of body functions that you've always relied on, loss of savings, loss of comforts. But I was still thankful. I was thankful that I had to deal with this spectre and not my kids, from a physical standpoint. And that day, I still had my house, my family, my friends and no one knows what tomorrow brings anyway. I didn't have the energy to start dreaming about Plan B, carefully crafting it in daydreams and thoughts. The well was dry.

And now, faced with a probable need for a Plan B, I was told that I should make a dreamboard. A woman came up to me after I had finally asked my question -- blurting it out before the moderator and other MomBosses could depart, "But what if you already had a dream that got taken away from you?" She slipped a card into my hand; she was a Life Coach. She said, "I have SO many ideas for you, right off the top of my head. Call me and we'll set up an appointment."

Sorry, lady, wherever you are. I didn't have time and I couldn't afford your consult fee. I needed to get home and use up the little energy I had left for the day and give it to my kids. Oh, and I was there that day for a free, fancy breakfast. And a morning out with a friend. And, NOW, lady -- I have to go start cutting out magazine pictures of things that would represent what I would want in the future? When all I wanted was to feel that feeling I had the day before my diagnosis. That the world was my oyster and if I worked REALLY, REALLY hard, I would make it someday. This was not a feeling sorry for myself thing as much as it was just another representation of feeling like I was running with a dry well. It was exasperating and scary.

When someone looks at a cancer patient and says, "How are you doing?? Is everything better now?" You know the answers in your head, but it really doesn't make for polite conversation. What you don't say is, "I'm really scared. I'm worried about the bills. How will we be able to afford college now? What if that lawyer really does take us to court? My medicine decreases my libido. I'm sad every time I look at where my breast used to be. I'm worried about my kids. I poop 18 times a day right now. I have a diaper bag in the car, packed in case I need it. We took more life insurance out on my husband than we did for me. Just what IS going on with the government and preexisting conditions? I can't control my emotions. The wheels are off the bus at home. We didn't know that my kid had Lyme Disease for five months. At the SAME EXACT time that people told you that you need to concentrate on yourself and the kids will be okay. I look young and able but it is REALLY HARD to go grocery shopping right now. We just spent our last $10 on gas for Tom to get to work today. Our two cars have 330,000 miles on them, collectively. How much longer will they last?"

I could go on and on, but what a cancer patient says is "Good, thanks. How was your vacation?" And the well-meaning person responds with, "Great! We needed to get away so much. I don't know how you do it. I'm just stressed doing my regular life! Let me know if you ever need anything!" I even had someone say to me, "I know you probably don't need anything, but if you ever do, let me know."

Later on in the year, I was able to pour myself into journaling, writing like it would save my life. But, that day? I was thankful for Judy, spring dresses, champagne mimosas, little waffles with mixed berries on top, tiny little quiches and petite yogurt cups. A treat for sure and a break from the everyday. And I said a prayer for the #MomBosses. They were obviously great moms and were living their truths. I just didn't know what my new truth could be at the time, I hadn't previously been in the market for one.

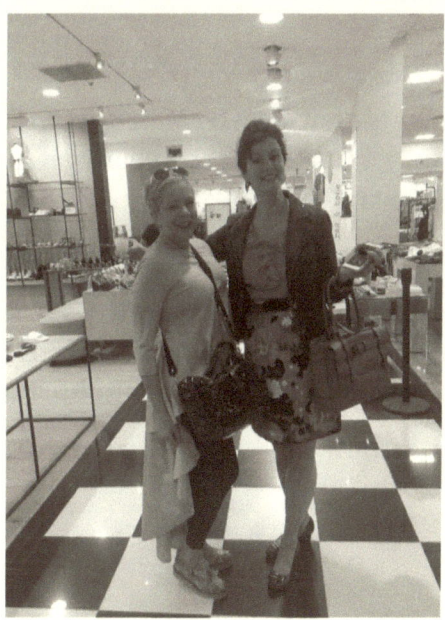

Targeted therapy infusion #16, June 11, 2018

Targeted therapy infusion #16 out of 18 and that's all I have to say about that. 88.88888888888...%

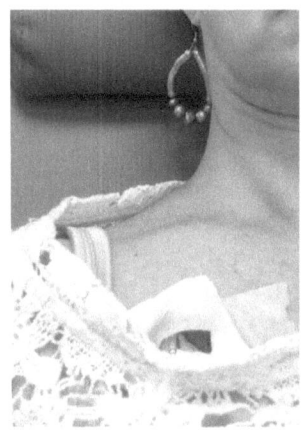

Jury Duty, June 13, 2018

Ok, Universe, Powers-that-be, the Man upstairs -- I'm ALL about doing my civic duty, but THIS is the year I get jury duty??? THIS ONE? This EXACT year??

In other news, it will be nice to bring home a paycheck again.

UPDATE: How often do you get to tell your kid that you are passing by his high school right now on a Sheriff's prisoner bus, on her way from the juror parking to the court house??

WAVE TO MOMMY, honey!!!!

* * *

THE HIGHS ARE GETTING HIGHER, THE LOWS AREN'T AS LOW

June 14, 2018

Collateral Damage

There is collateral damage when you are diagnosed with breast cancer. Actually, a diagnosis of any type of cancer brings collateral damage.

I'm not sure what to say when people say, "You're good now, right? You're done with chemo? The mastectomy? Radiation? You're good, right?"

The emotion of feeling "good" is subjective, it's relative, because the collateral damage is massive. There is no timeline to be followed. I am happy I no longer have to go through those big therapies, so that is "good," but there are SO many raw components left behind. The biggest blow to your self-esteem is how your body has changed on the outside. Never mind the mastectomy scar, you also now have a port scar. You have scars where tubes were put in your body. Your fingernails are not the same. They are paper thin, they peel. The medications cause joint pain. You have a lot of that in the morning. The radiation area has limited range of motion. I can no longer put my arm above my head without feeling like a muscle might rip.

It took me a little while to notice that my hot flashes are immediately preceded by a wave of nausea and the feeling of a panic attack about to hit. Now, I more and more frequently realize that I am about to ride the hot flash wave. I throw some peppermint essential oil on my neck along with the nearest ice pack. And never mind that the beauty requirement is now to have "on fleek" eyebrows. Huh? That ship has sailed...I will have to be satisfied with being "off fleek" and wait for my eyebrows to grow back in.

And that's just the outside. You listen when people say beauty is only skin deep. Or that beauty is in the eye of the beholder. And you believe this advice. You tell your children that every day. You dig deep to remember your self-esteem doesn't need anybody to approve of you. I once had a coworker tell me that my sweater, "does nothing for you." I started laughing at him. I asked him, "Oh, you thought I cared what you would think today when I put on this sweater?" Silly man. But I had a level of cockiness then. That's what a cancer diagnosis does to you. It strips you of your cockiness. Your happy-go-luckiness. Losing your cockiness and your happy-go-luckiness does not lend itself to being "good now." That's one of the things that goes through your mind when that beautiful loved one or friend is looking at you, the one you know loves you, hoping that you're "good now." Because you're still not good yet without those traits. And the word "inflammatory," a nasty component of my particular breast cancer, always gets me at my core fibers.

There's an anxiety there now, newly arrived in the last year since diagnosis. My heart goes out to people who have struggled their whole lives with anxiety and depression, I have a new understanding of it. And yet I don't. I know what caused mine. I can't imagine what it would feel like for someone to not know what causes theirs.

And chemo brain is a real thing. Tom and I might have a conversation that goes like this:

Me: Blah blah blah, um, that thing, it goes on the water? People ride on it?

Tom: A boat?

Me: Yes!!! A boat!!!

Chemo brain is a VERY REAL thing!! So you're navigating this road with the feeling of being less smart than you used to be.

There is the loss of pay, a year's salary, right in the prime of your life. The tripling, the quadrupling of medical bills.

Speaking of the prime of your life, there is the thought that you have raised your children, during which you have delayed gratification, to get to that point where you will have time with your spouse again, without interruption...whether it be conversation, peace, comfort. But instead of having more peace, there is even less than when you were taking care of the babies. There is the worry that you were so busy that you forgot "to live." That the kids don't know the family recipes. That your kids have only whispered their wishes to you; they haven't learned to scream their dreams.

I am quietly and trying oh-so-hard to let Tom NOT know that I'm guiding him through making the perfect smoothie for the kids. Or I might casually ask him, do you have the number of the pediatrician in your contacts? Even this morning -- I asked him to call our child in sick to school -- just to see if he knows the routine. By the way, he does. He is their dad. I've never been one to let someone get away with the statement, "Where are the kids? Is Tom babysitting them?" Um, no, you can't babysit your OWN kids. But, I quietly and for my own peace of mind, keep giving him these tests. Just in case. He pretends like he doesn't know what I'm doing. He's a good egg like that.

I have spent my whole career talking to my patients about the dangers of diet foods, processed foods, artificial anything. I have talked to them about getting their kids off high fructose corn syrup and artificial flavors. There is a worry that when I go back to work I will see the microglance that makes me know what just went through their head -- all of that didn't actually work for you, doc. This disease got me in my core values, my loves.

There is a part of John Steinbeck's book East of Eden that I think of often now. If memory serves me correctly, it was a conversation about getting over the loss of a loved one. And the advice was to, "act as if." Act AS IF everything is OK, keep putting one foot in front of the other and eventually, someday, there will be more good days than bad days. These days I am acting as if everything is good, while really not feeling all THAT good.

Waa, waa, waa. I'm assuming that if you read this far, you really do love and care about me. Or maybe this is giving you insight into a loved one that navigated this rocky road a lot more stoically than I. I hope I'm not giving away their magician's secrets. Listen, everybody has shit going on in their life. No one is guaranteed a shit-free life.

There's a quote that makes the rounds on Facebook that says, "Be kind. Many are fighting battles that you know nothing about." That's God's honest truth and I take it to heart. Because I'm not even getting into some of the deeper and deepest layers of my battle. It would invade people's privacies. My only hope is to give someone a glimmer, a reason to know, that although the big stuff is behind a cancer patient, they still might not be "good" yet. It was never your timeline. There are pieces to be picked up, with massively less stamina, increased anxiety and depression, less money and the feeling that you just don't feel good -- certainly not like yourself. And you miss that person you knew before.

You wonder and wonder about how to proceed. Vegan? Gluten free? No sugar? No alcohol? But then you reason with yourself.

What if this is my last hurrah? Should I be living life so strictly that champagne can't get in? A good oaky Chardonnay doesn't make the cut? Real, fresh whipped cream doesn't grace your lips? So, you end up reasoning, as my 91 year old grandmother likes to say, "Everything in moderation." Which is actually where I lived my whole adult life. So that stinks. There is NO conclusive answer to all of that wondering because I got cancer anyway.

A lot of people will tell you, "that which does not kill you makes you stronger." That's a favorite among your supporters. Affectionately, and I say this with absolute love, FUCK that. I was already strong enough. Please try not to say that to someone struggling.

I also no longer always think everything happens for a reason anymore. Shit happens. I was trying to follow a journal prompt the other day. WHAT IS YOUR FEELING RIGHT NOW? It took a few extra seconds to explore, but once I came up with it, I KNEW it intimately. I am impatient. IMPATIENT to get back to my real life.

But that's the lowest of the low stuff for now. And now for the highest of my highs, ANOTHER blessing from above -- the two amazing ladies at BeautifulSelf and their nonprofit organization focused on giving breast cancer fighters and survivors back their strength, beauty and confidence. It is a labor of love, what they do -- while looking like they are having the BEST TIME EVER. It is impossible not to get swept up into their stratospheric, meteoric atmosphere. It is impossible not to be having one of the best times of your life.

I have been on their waiting list since Halloween -- when I was still facing down more chemotherapy and the upcoming surgery. It sounded like a fun thing to shoot for, but I had no idea what I was in for. Jillian, a makeup ARTIST, that's all caps for a reason. Michele, a photographer that makes you feel like you're not being photographed. Their beautiful staff -- driving from Pennsylvania to get there for a breast cancer survivor photo shoot or getting a glimpse into lives as an observer, open to situations that you might not have experienced in your young life.

They were helping to make me FEEL again. I left their studio ready to take on the world. I literally felt like blowing stuff up. In a good way. The whole YOLO scene -- you only live once. But after having a year like I've had, the metamorphosis is underway. Thank you, LOVELY LADIES...you are not merely more angels on Earth that I've met post-7/7/17, you are extraordinary women to emulate. Judy, when you said that you found them in a Woman's Day magazine in the Morristown Memorial radiation waiting room and stood up and declared -- I HAVE TO FIND THEM. I know why now!! I'm putting a Beautiful Self tank top on my Christmas list. I am really excited about updating my profile picture. That hasn't been truth in advertising. That was when I had hair, about 9 months before diagnosis.

ISN'T IT AMAZING THAT I came up on their waiting list the same week that I decided to go back to work? I'm going back on Monday -- please give me extra berth, extra patience. I'm not totally ready, but I'm going to jump in head first anyway. You know, YOLO.

So, for now, I'm not "good now", but I'm working on it, acting "as if." But there is a marked difference; this is not the proverbial thin line. It is a big, fat, jagged line that you serpentine back and forth on. Because sometimes you forget what is actually going on and sometimes you don't. You have limitations you didn't have before along with being "off fleek" but I'm starting to catch a change in the atmosphere. It's like catching a few notes of a song that you used to know and you work really hard all day to remember what the song is, but you know the feeling it gave you then and it still gives you now.

* * *

BEAUTIFUL SELF
PHOTO SHOOT

June 14, 2018:

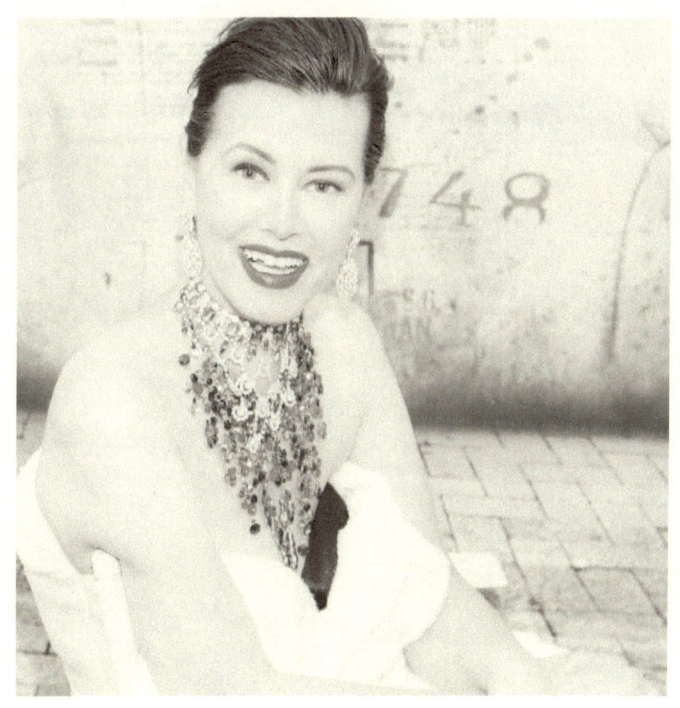

Dr. Shannon M. Mulvey

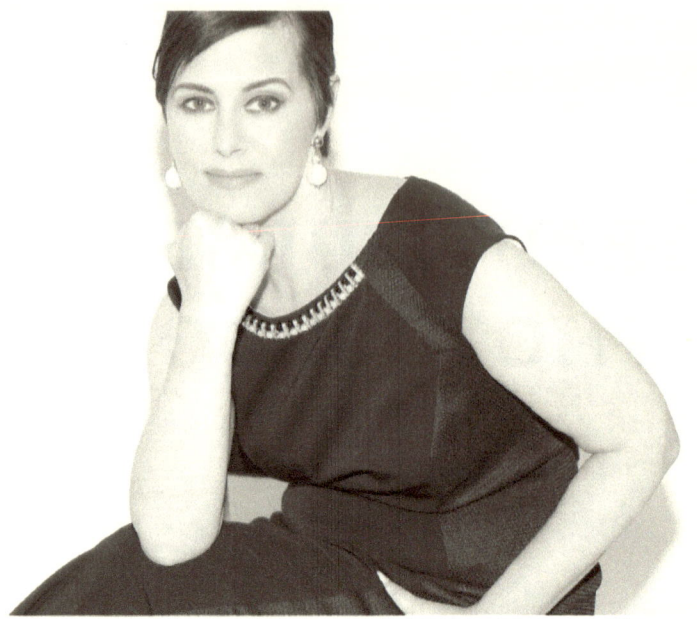

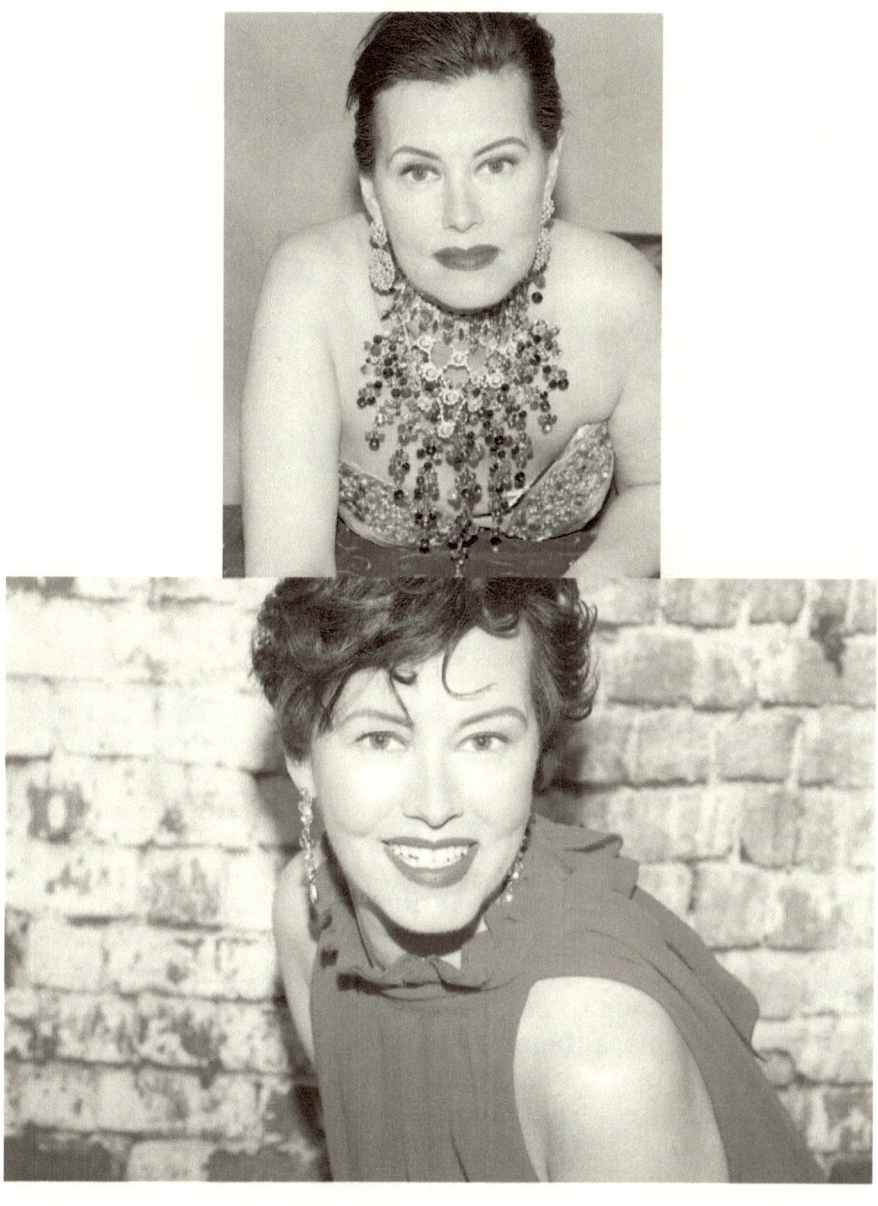

BIG INDUSTRY (TRIES) TO COME TO TOWN

June 26, 2018

Estrogen Mimickers

In 2016 and 2017, many of our town's residents got wind of a real estate deal that was proposed for our town. I'm no expert in the legal mumbo jumbo of municipal zoning, seemingly designed to confuse the average citizen on purpose. At its most simple, a chemical manufacturing plant was looking to set up shop in our tiny community. There were many hearings and ultimately the Planning Board voted down the application, despite the fact that it was an "approved use." Having already had to deal with an environmental cancer of unknown etiology, I took these hearings very seriously. I would go to each meeting, waiting to say my piece. I finally did get the opportunity on an early summer night. As of this date, the proposal remains in litigation, despite the opposition from the public and the Planning Board. Below, I have paraphrased some of what I stood up to say that night as my truth.

Last year, at the age of 45, I was diagnosed with Stage 3B inflammatory breast cancer. My only symptom was bruising of the breast which I attributed to my physical career as a chiropractor and my role as a mom. It wasn't hard to rationalize that I must have bumped it adjusting a patient at work or carrying a laundry basket at home. The cancer had already spread to my lymph nodes. It was found to be something called "Triple Positive." The part that concerns this chemical factory in my town is the fact that one of the hallmarks of my cancer concerns the hormone estrogen. I will come back to that.

Finding out this cancer news was the second worst day of my life. The WORST day of my life was telling my children, ages 14, 13, 10 and 8. My sons were leaving for Boy Scout camp the day after I found out and there was no way that I was going to dump this news on them before they left, for them to sort it out by themselves. I wanted to tell them where they felt safe to fall apart in their own home. We live about a mile from this proposed sight. I joined two ladies on my street who confided in me of their battles with breast cancer, one that occurred just four years ago. I joined two friends, each about a mile from here that battled cancer about ten years ago. These four women have 13 children between them.

When I found out the news, I was already familiar with the chemo and radiation routine. One of my best friends in town, age 48, had found out that she had cancer in the two years prior to my diagnosis and I had routinely accompanied her to her chemotherapy and radiation appointments. I knew the drill already and the fact that we both had to deal with cancer diagnoses in our 40s was a cruel joke.

Since my diagnosis, I have learned that within two square miles of my home, 17 people, mostly middle-aged, have been diagnosed with cancer in recent years. We have 47 children between us. You have NO idea the pain caused by cancer until you've had to tell your children that you have it.

My cancer is estrogen driven. It eats estrogen like candy. Estrogen fans it's flames. Why is this important? Because artificial fragrance is a known estrogen mimicker. Every time I am exposed to artificial fragrance or chemicals, my cancer would want to eat it. Of the approximately 1500 chemicals that this company is using, many are carcinogenic. Estrogen mimickers tend to do that in a body. I would assume that many are banned in socialist countries where they country pays for their citizens' healthcare.

This road is already the site of past contamination from pharmaceutical manufacturing. Maybe we would like to say they didn't know any better then. But we can't say that now. We KNOW better and once you know, you can't unknow. If we KNOW better, then we need to DO better and we can NOT make this about a tax benefit. 47 children in this one mile circumference that I even know of this year. How would you like 47 more next year? How would putting these synthetic fragrances into our surrounding towns affect that number the following year?

I know one thing to be true. Each and every time I tell a provider that I don't have the breast cancer gene and I have zero out of twelve risk factors for breast cancer, they all say the same thing. What they say is, "It must be environmental."

The more I say that my town of 2.59 square miles wants to put a chemical factory in it, the more absurd it sounds. It should sound absurd to you. Especially if we start talking tax benefits as it's redeeming quality. You know what they are doing in the more prosperous towns around this area? They are learning how to take care of their town fields without pesticides. They are looking into safer surroundings for their kids. It sounds like this town is trying to do the opposite.

How many of our town's children would have to be affected for it to be meaningful to anyone? As I ponder this town's and this chemical factory's intentions, 47 town children do not appear to be enough.

If I sound angry about this, it's because I am. If you're not angry about this, it's only because it hasn't hit your family yet. But when it does, you will be angry, too. Especially when you figure out that there was a choice that was made to bring us to that place in time.

I'm not sure what the average age of the planning board is. But the average age of people I know with cancer right now is 45. If you didn't know 18 people that had cancer with an average age of 45 when you were my age, you are very lucky. But that IS the case now and the environment plays a massive role. Hopefully it hasn't hit your children yet or your grandchildren's lives yet, but at this rate, it's just a matter of time. I wouldn't have thought it either a year ago today.

ONE YEAR AGO TOMORROW

July 6, 2018

The Mammogram

A year ago tomorrow, I walked out of work on a beautiful summer Friday. I think I was originally supposed to work that afternoon. But I had spent the morning and the day before trying to secure an appointment for a mammogram. Some of the places gave me appointments for September. For some of the offices, they didn't answer and the staff never called me back. But one mammography office was able to get me in that afternoon.

I walked out of work and I remember yelling over my shoulder, "Bye, guys!! I'm going to my mammography appointment now! Have a great weekend and I'll see you Tuesday!" We had a little joke at work. I always said, "Ladies?" And when I would say that, they would respond, "All the ladies." A la Salt-N-Pepa, circa 1991. When I was twenty years-old and they were just being born. But I'm sure I probably threw in the word "ladies" that day;

I almost always did.

I had time to kill before my appointment and I decided to treat myself to the Green Goddess salad at Panera Bread. I probably scrolled Facebook while I ate. It was still new and shiny then and I hadn't seen any assholes spew their opinions yet, as if anyone cares about anyone else's opinions except their own. You know the type. It is easy to separate Facebook posts and probably even people into two groups. Those that have something to say and those that say something but with the intention of you learning something they ACTUALLY wanted you to know about them. If that's still unclear, it might sound something like this, "OF COURSE I will make the cupcakes for the school party, but I just have to swing by my 10 bedroom beach house on the beach in the Hamptons first." In any case, the day still had promise.

Even going in for the appointment, I felt OK. Big, fluffy, white robe, ladies sitting around reading magazines. I brought a book with me that day. I thought it would be a great opportunity to start a new one. It was called The River at Night and it was about four women in their "middle years" doing something super courageous and brave, setting out on a camping and white water rafting trip. That would not be first or even one hundredth on my list of things I'd like to do, but I was looking forward to the read and being inspired to make some courageous plans of my own, also being a woman of a certain "middle" age.

After the mammogram, they asked me to have a seat and wait. I started that book again, wrapped up in my spa-like robe. That's what I kept doing that afternoon. Starting the book again, I couldn't concentrate for some reason. They asked me to come back in after a few minutes just to check some things out.

That wasn't what did me in. What did me in was the multiple faces at the doctors' and nurses' desks that all looked up at me when I walked back in. It felt suspect. Their faces all popped up in unison. It was like realizing that people are talking about you, but you have no proof. More pictures were taken; they asked me to go sit and wait again. And I started that book again. And again. And again.

They called me back in. A doctor walked in that had read the films. He said, "We have found something, a couple of things, in fact." My first thought was to ask something I had learned a long time ago in a radiology class in chiropractic school. I just knew you wanted a capsule around those tumors. You want a spatula to go in and lift it out like a hard-boiled, future Easter egg. I asked, "Are they encapsulated?" I knew he was sorry to tell me that they were not. I could tell by his face.

At 4:27 that afternoon, I sent a text to Tom, my mother and my sister. I still have it. It reads, "It's not good. There's a mass. I'm getting changed and need to meet with the nurse. I'll call you as soon as I can."

And then, a second text, "I'm shaking -- it's 2" big, there's a lymph node, too. I have to come back Monday for a needle biopsy using ultrasound. Meeting with nurse now to set up Monday appointment, irregular borders and he said to prepare myself -- probably 70 percent malignant." You know why I texted it, right? Because I ABSOLUTELY couldn't speak it. It's why I was not good about returning calls this year. It's why I relied on texting to make connections with you. They were lifelines to me, but I COULD NOT verbalize anything to any of you I was already over the edge.

My life changed in that room. My kids' lives changed in that room. My and Tom's "For Better or For Worse" vows took on a surreal meaning as to what "for worse" actually meant. I'm so glad I didn't know that kind of stuff on my wedding day. You think it's just something traditional to say that day, but someday it might mean that nightmares can come true.

That was the last day that I was at work for almost an entire year. I am happy to say that I went back two weeks ago. I cried all the way there. It was SO super emotional. I cried when I walked in and when I saw each one of the "ladies, all the ladies."

The men, too, but I have nothing to call their subgrouping.

Truth be told, I am not the same. I'm not the same person, physically or mentally, so that loss is noticeable. But, boy was I happy to pull myself up to my beautiful desk, turn on my computer and walk in to see my first patient in my most favorite office that I've ever worked, albeit 50 weeks later. I am again working a half day today, but I'm not going to pass by Panera Bread on my way home and I'm definitely not making ANY fucking appointments for this afternoon.

There is something special in my head to say that I was "only" out for 50 weeks, not a full year. And, in this middle aged, middle class cancer of mine -- trust me -- you NEVER want to lose a year of your salary AND, as I was so kindly reminded yesterday by financial men in suits, a whole year's 401K contributions, at exactly the wrong time.

Getting back to work after 50 weeks has been just like riding a bicycle. Underwater. A bicycle you are riding underwater. But all the mechanics work the same and you're still moving forward. Some of the patients looked at me like I was the new one here on that first day back. One made the comment, "it must be nice to take a year off." No way. I wouldn't have chosen it this way, lady. But I've been here 15 years, now tell me about you.

I'm going to pass through 7/7/18 quietly -- but the words YEAR ONE down, 54 to go, will most certainly be on a loop in my head, a welcome skipping of the record. It would have been hard to fathom that same time, last year...but today is already different. There were terrible storms that morning and my kids' swim team practice was cancelled. Terrible storms are forecast for today and swim team was able to be held. See? Already different. And I'm sitting at my desk, working, with nothing to do for later this afternoon, nowhere to be and that sounds like a gift from above.

One more infusion to go. The 18th out of 18, I'm coming for you...

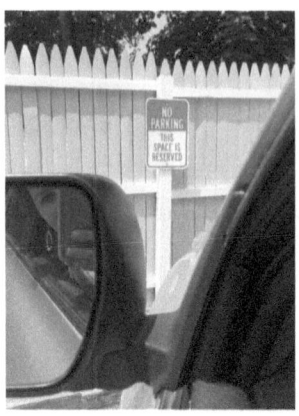

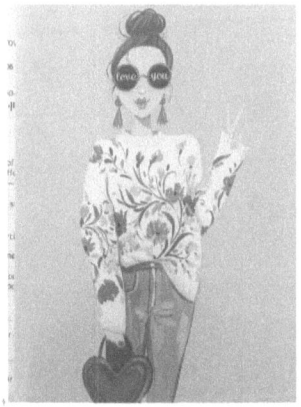

THE LAST INFUSION

July 23, 2018

I'm OUTTA here!!

I'm always impressed by the people that finish cancer therapy and they're smiling. Ringing the bell, saying goodbyes to the friends they made. People who take pictures of themselves smiling in their chemotherapy chair. There's a real, "I've got this" attitude. I don't have that as I finish my last infusion today. Eighteen out of eighteen. I'm sorry that I don't. I wish that I did. I feel like I'm letting people down when I don't act thrilled. Instead, my attitude today is: "Fuck you. Don't ever do that to me again, motherfucker." I don't know to whom to direct this sad attitude. Not my family and friends, of course. Not towards myself, although there is an element that says -- I took care of my body, so why didn't it take care of me? Lots of yinning over here over the years; I thought there was enough banked to be able to yang. But maybe it's hard to undo all of the Hawaiian Punch I drank through college. YUCK! I surely don't direct it towards God. I took the poem Footprints very much to heart this year. I am EXTREMELY aware that I was being carried for a long time. There were only two footprints in the sand for me this year. Not mine. Every day I'm thankful for that. I don't direct it towards my providers although they did not see the best side of me. They have no idea what my real personality is like. So I have this undirected fuck you-ness that needs to get resolved. Don't worry about me on that aspect. I have been journaling like crazy. Three pages every morning. Does anyone else wake up with that feeling of angst? Of all the things that you need to do today? I didn't used to. I used to wake up with a feeling of excitement, but I am realizing that it is almost the same feeling. So getting to that journal has been sort of a brain dump -- to get to the good stuff, let's address the bad stuff and leave it in that pretty little pink book, then I can get on with the day. I even take the time to go back in and circle the negative stuff I write and try to write in pretty Sharpie colors in the margins a positive way to spin the crappiness I sometimes write about. Positive affirmations, if you will. So that's helping a ton. I'm sure that when I can look down and see something familiar there, that will help. In due time. But I still need to be waiting on that because of the whole "inflammatory" aspect.

These are lessons in patience. We all have them every day. I just never expected one to last years.

I am only one year out. And I obviously still have anger over the whole thing. But I also wrote in my journal this week that I wish I could send a postcard from today back to myself a year ago. Because this morning I woke up with peace, I have learned what love is this year and I am still alive. It was a beautiful morning (to me). I had a hot cup of tea. I had a plan for the day. I have returned to work in the last couple of weeks. My hair has grown back in. I have a fresh pedicure on my toes. And miracles are occurring every day. There is fun to be had again! Monday night I spent with best friends and the Foo Fighters. When I got the tickets last November, I could barely walk from the chemo effects. I've already talked about that ad nauseum. But I danced and screamed and cried and sang for three straight hours on Monday night. I wouldn't have been able to do that at different points this past year. This week I could. Tears flung off the sides of my face as I heard the songs that got me through this year...it was SO emotional...

Best of You:

Is someone getting the best, the best, the best of you?

Has someone taken your faith?

It's real, the pain you feel,

You trust, you must confess

The life, the love

You die to heal

The hope that starts the broken hearts

You trust, you must confess...

And then, this one:

Times Like These:

It's times like these you learn to live again...to give and give again, learn to love again, time and time again.

I, I'm a new day rising

I'm a brand new sky

To hang the stars upon tonight...

But this one, THIS ONE flung my tears...

Walk

Learning to walk again

I believe I've waited long enough

Where do I begin?

Now, for the very first time,

Don't you pay no mind

Set me free, again

To keep alive, a moment at a time

That's still inside, a whisper to a riot

The sacrifice, the knowing to survive,

The first decline, another state of mind

I'm on my knees, praying for a sign

Forever, whenever, I never wanna die...

I'm dancing on my grave,

I'm running through the fire

I never wanna die

I never wanna leave

I'll never say goodbye

These primal screams on Monday night did me good. And then, as always to end the Foo night — *Everlong*...

And I wonder, when I sing along with you,

If everything could ever feel this real forever...

If anything could ever be this good again...

More fun? Taylor Swift gave free tickets to the Girl Scouts of Northern New Jersey for her concert this weekend and I was able to bring Claire to her first ever concert. She is a MEGA Swiftie. And I got to surprise her with free tickets. More singing and dancing to be had!! And another reminder to SHAKE IT OFF!

I'm not going to ring a bell. I will probably do the "Irish goodbye." That totally goes against my grain but I just don't feel like celebrating.

I will say a prayer for the people there, for both the patients and the caretakers. I know I'll see them again. I know that prescriptions will be written, follow-ups will take place -- I might even make a crazy call when I am afraid that a seemingly unrelated symptom might be signs of a return. But that is hard to imagine. I never had any symptoms in the first place.

I will also take one last look at the "Wall of Hope" chalkboard that I always checked in on at every one of my chemotherapy and/or infusion sessions. Maybe I'll even leave a message.

And today the feeling is this: when I'm done, I will pick myself up off the ground, dust myself off, straighten my clothes, pat down stray hairs. Look around to see if anyone saw anything, adjust that crown, reapply some lipstick. And walk out with my head held high. You never saw me here.

Next up, port removal, a minor procedure, all things considered. More medications...

Tom took off this afternoon to accompany me. We will surely drink champagne though. Not because #18 is finito, but because it's going to be just an average Monday afternoon after that appointment. Today, I would like to raise a toast to "average." It's totally underrated. Believe you ME.

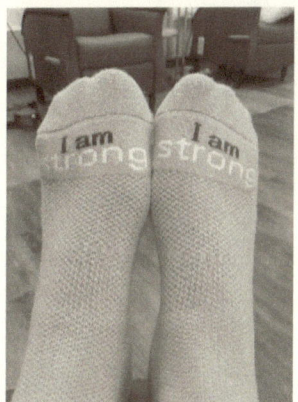
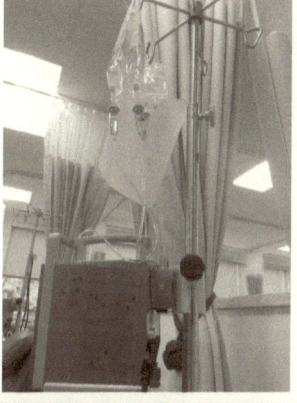

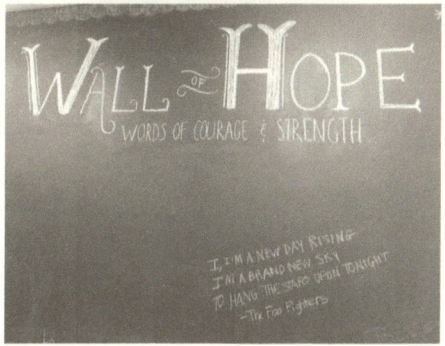

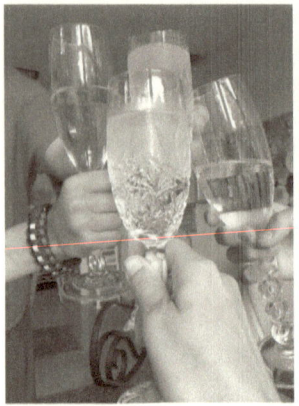

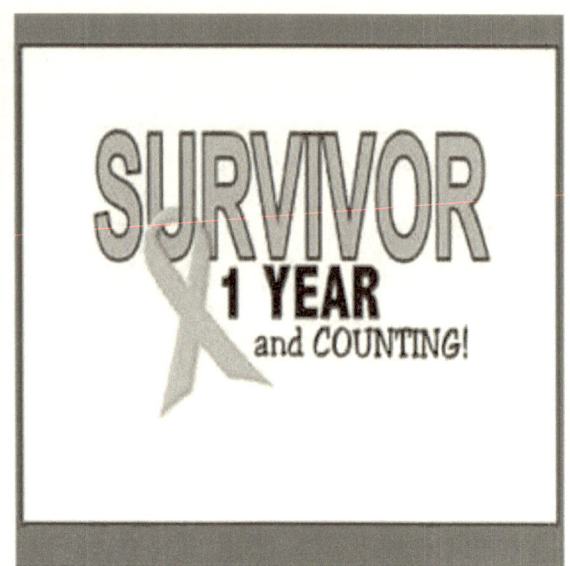

THE PORT IS OUT

August 3, 2018

Back to the OR, STAT!
GET THIS THING OUT!!

This port of mine is out. A minor procedure, as these things go. I was still in the operating room but there was no general anesthesia, like there was for it's placement. Locals only! Said placement was one year and two days ago. First chemo was one year and one day ago. I guess that's why it literally feels like it has been a year and a day. Because it was. There are lots of congratulations being flung at me. I am sincerely thankful, but the only way I can equate it to something that might be meaningful is this way. Getting it out is like being given a vacuum cleaner or an iron for your birthday and the giver is expecting you to be happy about it. Well — you could certainly use a vacuum cleaner. You might be mildly interested in the suction that your new vacuum has as opposed to your old vacuum. But it's just a passing fancy. You never wanted a new vacuum. And for the record, I don't need an iron. I have a beautiful one. It has all the bells and whistles. It is perfect. I got it exactly 29 years ago when I left for college, August of 1989. So don't worry about giving me an iron. I think I've used it two or three times now. I'm probably an expert and it's just waiting for me to put it to use!

The first time my children ever stayed in a hotel room that was memorable, Sam and Zach ran through it, yelling and screaming. I should probably say they ran across. Probably took them .2 seconds. They absolutely could not believe that we had a refrigerator in our room. And a TV. This was like living in the lap of luxury for them. But when Sam took down the ironing board from behind the door, put it on the floor and with that twinkle in his eye that Sam always has, exclaimed, "And look what else they left us! They left us a surfboard!", I knew I was in trouble. And he got on that ironing board/surfboard and posed his very best Beach Boys pose. It made Tom want to throw a quiz question at them. He picked up the iron and asked them if they knew what THAT was. And one of them said, "That's a sewing machine." The other one said, "Definitely. That is definitely a sewing machine." To date, at least three of my children got that question wrong on their Kindergarten first sounds tests. That iron remains elusive for them. And I'm thinking it will remain so -- they are just going to have to memorize that it starts with an "I".

There has been a love-hate relationship with this port-thing. Tom actually wanted me to ask for it, wanted me to bring it home and he said he was going to take great pleasure in smashing it with a sledgehammer. However, I was not allowed to take it home. I keep thinking about what a survivor/thriver said to me recently about hers. She said that she has only love for her port. She looks at it like it saved her life. So I get that, too. But now I'm wondering if she meant the libation?

I was even a little worried about having it taken out. What if? That old question. But it turns out the new thinking is that because it's a foreign body, it needs to come out if not being used. The nurse even walked me through the thought process. It is literally sclerosing my veins while it's there. And she said I was still young enough for my veins to heal. Okay, veins, I'm doing this for you. Don't say I never cared about you. And I'm figuring, if I ever needed one again, having it replaced wouldn't be my worst problem. There would be bigger fish to fry at that moment in time but I'm not going to go further than that. Not today. I never really did get to the point where I wasn't aware of its presence. Lying face down, I felt it. Passenger side seat belts bothered it. I hate ending sentences with a preposition but I don't feel like changing it. Nor changing that one, either. Bathing suit straps bothered it, too. Max's head seemed to make contact with it fairly regularly when he came in for one of his gigantic hugs. Farewell, port! Another item to check off the list of things to do.

Are you a risk taker? Can you throw it all to the wind and live with the results? Have risks paid off for you? Did your wildest dreams come true? I used to be like that, but I'm not a risk taker any more. Slow and steady wins the race over by me. I miss that carefree, devil-may-care attitude but it's been nice not to feel the need to respond to every passing whim/opportunity/danger that comes my way. I guess that's what comes with age, the ability to discern between good risks and bad risks, good dreams and bad, wild child antics and middle-aged comforts. So imagine my surprise when I came across the risks of this Inflammatory Breast Cancer diagnosis. It took me down a dark tunnel this week. This is going to be a real risky thing to navigate. Because IBC only affects 1-3% of breast cancer women (some say 1-5%), it's really LOW risk to end up with. In fact, it is unusual to see more than one in a family. It is hard to be seen in mammograms. Just the very definition of IBC guarantees that you are most likely already Stage 3 or 4 by the time anyone knows anything. Check! There is a guaranteed mastectomy coming your way and chemotherapy will almost always precede the surgery. Check, check! Simply because it reduces the skin involvement, so the surgeon doesn't have to deal with that area unless healthier. The follow-up radiation is intense to get rid of the "nests" of bad cells. All of this can sound very similar to a typical breast cancer but it's not, simply because of its survivability. It is almost always in women and tends to occur at a younger age. Check and check. Risk DECLINES with higher education. WHENEVER you read about IBC the word "aggressive" is ALWAYS used. And here is where it diverges from the more typical breast cancers. The median survival rate is 57 months. That is NOT alot.

Before chemotherapy was introduced as a therapy to combat IBC, it had a 2 percent, five-year survival rate. With chemotherapy it has been "revolutionized" to 40 percent. That's the word currently being used. I hate when people say I picked an easy cancer to get and I do hear that. Or I hear something like this, "Well, you could get run over by a car today just stepping out of your house." Well, I know that. That is the truth. But this feels similar to finding out there's a car actually out looking for you in your neighborhood. Vigilance is mandatory and necessary.

I know I am not a statistic. I am not a number. I was recently asked if I regretted eating organic all these years or following a healthy lifestyle. As IF. I am looking at it like — maybe this is giving me my good results. What if I had gotten it at a younger age? What if, literally a year and a day later, I wasn't sitting in my favorite chair drinking a cup of tea right now?

It is interesting. There are plenty of 90-year-old grandparents around. I have read that the reason why they're still kicking so lively is because they DID have an organic diet as kids. They WERE breastfed. They were NOT on every medication in the world. They had more outdoor playtime. Processed foods? They had no place in their homes. The industrial age changed all of that and we have seen how it has affected our states of health. I can only hope that I was able to swing that pendulum back in my family, hopefully giving them better outcomes in their lives. I had the good fortune of teaching 350 natural childbirth couples over the years. Literally 700 people spiraled in and out of my living room for 10-12 weeks each. Every size, shape, race, economic class and denomination you could imagine came through. I even had religious men sitting at my kitchen table, reading the Torah, while Tom cleaned up the dishes from dinner. I was not shy about telling ANY of them healthier ways to feed their children. I thought of it like planting seeds. I'm hoping those seeds have lead to better choices in A LOT of people who are in charge of A LOT of little people. Back to my original thesis. Once you know? You can't unknow.

A cheat sheet might look like this, vegetables and fruits = good. Ingredients you can't pronounce = bad. Got it?

Right now, I am looking at three days of not being able to get the area wet, two weeks of not being able to soak. That sort of stinks this time of year. But the whole year stunk. So, let's get it all over with. It's the same reasoning I ended up with four kids close in age together. If I had the chance to see life out of their diapers? I might not have gone back. And my little guy's head knocking on that port of mine, every single time, would not have reminded me of what I am fighting for this year. Next year? I'll be fighting for a vacation. #TRUTH

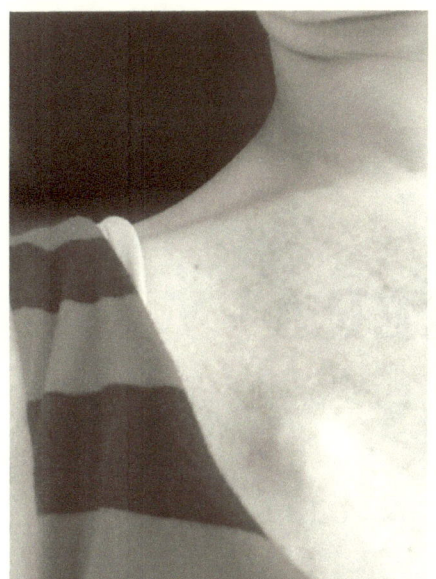
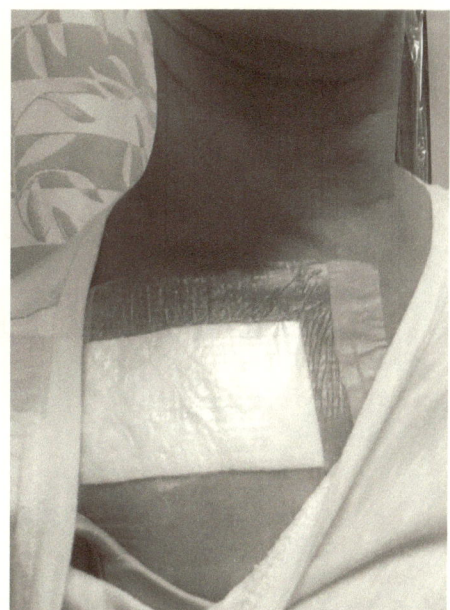

ORAL CHEMOTHERAPY

September 26, 2018

Shit.

"Just when I thought I was out, they pull me back in."

Shitshow. Shithead. Shitola. Shit. Shit. Shit. Shit. Shit. Shit. I didn't have time for a new hobby. It's too embarrassing to even talk about but this is the next chapter. The shit chapter. It's a little crude. And if you're sensitive, move to the next Facebook post. But let's just back the hell up first.

It's been a shitstorm getting the kids back to school at the same time as working. I went back to work during the last weeks of school last year. So I had a whole summer of getting used to working again. But having to put the career back together with the school year has not been easy. I feel like I am either working or resting; there is no in between. We actually forgot about a picture day this week. My former self gets annoyed at my present self over stuff like that. I just keep losing ground on that list of things to do and there are some really important things on it, too. And it's deceptive because I am past a lot of the bigger things on my "cancer" list of things to do. But there was always another big item coming on that shitlist of mine; I've alluded to it in the past. And it's now arrived. Oh, shit!

My oncologist didn't even want to prescribe this new medicine. He said that he almost never did because the side effects were so dastardly. Especially after a year like I've had. He felt bad about it, even. We sat there in his office and he told me this is what he would do for his wife, for his mother, for his sister, if they had my diagnosis. Those are magic words to me. I always want to know what someone would do for their own family. So this medicine comes from a specialty pharmacy. You just can't walk into your local pharmacy. It comes with lessons. A nurse calls you. A pharmacist calls you. It comes FedExed to you. It comes with a SUPPORT KIT. It costs $11,000 a MONTH. But you might be able to pay a $10 co-pay. Neither of those are typos, they both have the right amount of zeros. But all of that remains to be seen. I've seen that the amount billed will be $11,000. I haven't seen the insurance billing of it yet. But it does make me wonder why they won't cover a wig.

At my very first visit with the oncologist, it's one of the first drugs he brought up as miraculous for me. But then he sort of sat on it for many months. I had to get past all of the other therapies first. We had talked about it a couple of times, but the last time I went in there, he had a piece of very good news. The full dose is six pills a day. Women who started at that dose sometimes had a very, very, very hard time. He told me that he had seen great results with starting at two pills a day for a week. Then adding one pill each week, until you eventually get to six per day. So that was the new plan. It does add to the end date. I figured it out the other day, it adds 11 to 12 more days to the original treatment plan of 365 days. That autumn solstice of 2019 will be a happy day for me. I know it seems like this month should've been about pulling it all together, post port removal and everything.

It IS this month, except it's next year's September. September of 2019. Patience AIN'T my thing.

The bottle had been sitting in my kitchen cabinet for about three weeks. I would see it whenever I opened the door. We had a real cat and mouse game going on. There was no way I was starting it at the end of summer. I won that battle. But I was still the mouse. There was no way I was starting it before Labor Day weekend; we were heading to the beach. Shannon, 2, Cat, 0. And then we had a couple of fun things to celebrate the following week and there was no way I was going to be down for the count for them (4,0). I didn't really want to start it for the first day of school (5,0). So I had my calendar circled to start it on September 10th. Monday. Every Monday is New Year's Day to me, new resolutions get made every week. It always has been.

I even had to join a Facebook group -- a closed, secret group where women can opine about these mischievous side effects. What I read wasn't pretty. It made me keep putting off that start date. These are not possible side effects. These are probable side effects. Many women stop taking it; many women talk about stopping it as a quality-of-life issue; many have ended up in the hospital. But the more I thought about it, and I really had to take time to wrap my head around this, the more I had to look at it like the gift I was giving myself for my 47th birthday. And my 48th birthday. And all of the other birthdays. Because I will be taking it for 365+ days. So the plan was to start it four days after my birthday. Now I was the cat and it was the mouse. Here is what the gift is to myself. Why I am going to at least attempt to take it for the full prescribed year, over chasing better quality-of-life issues. Whatever my rate of survivability is right now, and I truly forget what it is (maybe I try to forget), but it increases THAT number by 34 percent. And you just don't always see that in the oncology world. I am jumping through that golden ring. Because I'm spooked by that "40 percent survivability at five years" statistic of inflammatory breast cancer. I'm not capitalizing that proper noun because I don't want to give it any power. That 34 percent increase on top of the baseline rate, that one's MINE and one thing's for sure. I am stocked up on probiotics. And REALLY soft paper products. So far, so good. Today is day 18. They say day 8 is the really tough one. And it was.

Here is the other reason why this drug is important for me. Out of everything I've medically done this past year, and it's been A LOT — none of these medicines have crossed my blood brain barrier. And this one does. What does that mean? We've always known this cancer would be more likely to go to my bones or my brain or my organs faster than it would ever get to my other breast. Another reason why I opted for a single mastectomy. (Side note: remember how I once said that my dictation of mastectomy always auto corrected to mystic to me? Now it just autocorrected to misstep to me.) So, just in case some cells slipped out and got to my brain or anywhere else, this is the one drug that crosses the blood brain barrier. And can zap any potential cancer cells lurking there before they could make themselves known. Anyway, that is the dream AND the plan. I am particularly taken with that quote lately, "dreams without plans are just wishes." Or something like that.

So now I had the plan. I had put it on the calendar. I had marked it "D-day." With absolutely no wish to equate my meaning of it with the actual D-Day. Because my "D" means something totally different. So there it was, set for Monday the 10th. I even picked the time. 2 o'clock. Before the kids came home from school, if I was home. While I'm on my lunch hour, if I'm at work. I put an alarm in my phone, 2:00 daily. Ok, A PLAN IS A PLAN.

But the day before that, I was signed up for a six-hour continuing education seminar. I thought I would get some credits out of the way; I have a lot of making up to do this year. And I took these pills with me. I threw them in my bag. I knew they were there the whole day. The lecture was incredibly interesting. Women's Health Issues. I'm all over that. Sign me up for that any day over something like the "Overview of an Adolescent

Elbow and its Relationship to Playing Sports." I actually just made that lecture name up. But that's how dry they sometimes sound to me. As for the lecture I was sitting in last Sunday, the person running it was brilliant. He knew his stuff. We spent a lot of time talking about "Methylation." If you're interested? Look it up. But here's the deal. You are constantly -- and at any moment in time -- and especially when you procreate -- a product of every single thing that has ever happened to you or has been put into your body or lived in the environment in your past. Scary, right? That's how somebody without a family history of, or risk factors for, can get breast cancer. It's why bad things can happen to good people. And it really all comes down to inflammation. The top three health killers -- heart disease, stroke and cancer, are caused by inflammation. That doesn't mean to start taking an anti-inflammatory. It means to stop putting inflammatory things into yourself or surrounding yourself with them. And start boycotting the companies that make them.

The lecturer was not a doomsdayer, however. He had a funny attitude. He made a comment like, "What do you want? Do you want to live to 30 or 40 and be a caveman or do you want to live to 80 or 90 in a dirty world? You pick." So my philosophy on getting through this has been to pick the best of the Western medicine and the best of the Eastern medicine, to bring a lot of my holistic things into my plan and a lot of good common sense. Common sense tells me that I will keep eating my organic fruits and vegetables, exercising "moderately" and you don't have to tell me THAT twice. I have never been a "contenda." My vitamin pile is ridiculous. I sent myself for bloodwork and I now know exactly what is going on. I will keep journaling, I will keep sleeping. But it turns out that one isn't a choice. Fatigue is one of the biggest side effects of this new drug and one I'm already feeling. Again. It's why I am not getting back to anybody. It's why I'm not out much. It stinks to have been down the tunnel for over a year and to finally feel like I could get out and smell the flowers and then to suddenly be back feeling this kind of fatigue.

Ugh. It's not welcome here. But a necessary evil this year nonetheless. My new bedtime is 8:30, which particularly stinks since I get home from work at 8:00.

I related a couple of months ago that I had not been able to bring myself to clean out my bra drawer. I still haven't. Well, I'm doing it ASAP. This week!! And here's the reason why. I just became aware of a foundation that distributes necessities to homeless people in both New York City and New Jersey. Necessities like bras. And they are located one town away. I know there are a lot of worthy causes to donate your clothes to, but if any women want to pull out those bras and send them my way, I will happily deliver (hopefully a ton of) bras to this foundation in October. Leave them by my door!! Or send them to me!

Incidentally and unrelatedly, some of you sidle up to me. You get a little close. That's OK; I don't have a bubble. But you look around to make sure nobody can hear you and then when you think nobody can, you ask me if I have thought about getting my medical marijuana card. It's sort of funny. For the record, I did get my medical marijuana card. I am a card carrying member. I originally thought it would help me with my chemotherapy side effects. I made a journey to Montclair one day. All I could think of is that my Girl Scout troop should set up their cookie sales right outside that dispensary. I took it exactly twice. It did not go well. It did not help my side effects like I thought it could. Even though there is massive evidence that cannabis can help shrink cancer tumors, and it really, really can, it can actually have the opposite effect on my type of cancer. Because mine was estrogen-based, some of the aspects of medical marijuana actually can make an estrogenic cancer tumor grow. Never mind the Tamoxifen. If a drug is made less useful by eating grapefruit, as Tamoxifen is, cannabis can have a similar effect -- it makes the Tamoxifen less useful. And I need it to be useful right now. Very, very useful. But, no. I won't make a trip to a dispensary to get it for you. I'm too busy sleeping.

As for the other massive side effect, the really, really bad one, I'm not even going to talk about that one. I'm going to have to let you guess that one. Sorry, some things are just going to have to be left private. I'm a lady. I'm sorry if you think that's shitty of me for not talking about it more, explaining it more. Truly. Shit. I feel terrible. But I know you'd be a good listener if I did.

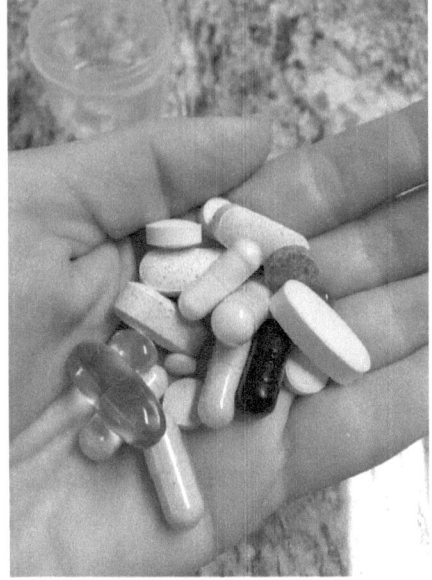

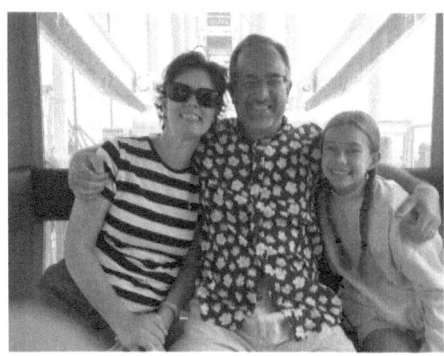

BRASSIERES FROM MY BOSOM BUDDIES

November 3, 2018

Brassieres

Brassieres -- "As an aside on the way words can shift in meaning over time and between languages, a brassière in modern French most commonly refers to a baby's vest (in the British sense of an undershirt) or to a lifebelt, while the usual word for a bra in that language is soutien-gorge, literally a bosom support", at least according to World Wide Words -- which is the first thing that popped up when I searched "Word for bras." Who knew?

I'm pretty sure one of husband's former dreams came true. Bras, bras and more bras started showing up on our doorstep. It may be the dreams of my teenage sons, as well although I'll never ask and they didn't seem to notice packages by the front door. But they don't notice full garbage cans to take out or laundry piles to put away, so I think we're all safe. Who DID notice? Little Max. Who, more than a couple of times yelled out, "Look! Someone left us a package." A simple reply, "They are bras to donate," led to a very dramatic scene of him screaming, dropping the bag and running away as fast and as far as he could.

That being said, when September came and I STILL had not cleaned out the "soutien-gorges" from my drawer -- the ones that no longer made sense post left simple mastectomy, I became inspired. I saw that a drive was being done during October by a continuing education company at which I sometimes take continuing education credits to collect bras for homeless women. Bras turn out to be a MAJOR necessity for homeless women and I thought -- well, maybe THAT will get my derrière into gear and cleaning out that drawer.

I had made a feeble attempt one day during the summer. It was a day that I also had to donate favorite bathing suits and buy mastectomy bathing suits. I saw the bras in there but the bathing suit day was still fresh in my mind. I returned to the job after seeing this drive. It still wasn't a stellar day when I tried again. Minds attached to intact bodies REALLY do feel like you can lose a breast and live. You can't always lose an organ and live. So it may seem like an easy decision and they are right. It's an easy decision but it will always be sad to face myself in the mirror. Nobody likes to be disfigured, whether it can be seen around your clothes or not.

To motivate myself, I let people know that I would be collecting the bras during the month of October. I put it in one of my last posts. A little while later, I added it to our private town Facebook page. I did this almost as an afterthought. Then I told my coworkers. But lo and behold, bags of bras started showing up everywhere. On the porch, in front of the garage, on my desk at work. My meager attempts to clean that drawer out became bolder and I tried again. And yet, still more showed up. People yelled to me from across bonfires that they had more. And at cocktail parties. Some showed up in my veggie co-op basket returns.

As difficult as it has been to part with them, it has been JUST as difficult to attain the supposedly FREE mastectomy ones that I am entitled to as one of my "benefits" from my insurance company. I will probably never use the words "insurance benefits" together in a sentence again. You've probably seen that married duo used by me for the last time. They always feel like they are actually estranged from each other. And that's because of DIFFERENT stories for another time. But one day, I actually found myself sitting on hold for the approximately 3-4 hours it took for the insurance company to ascertain that -- YES -- I am ENTITLED to FREE MASTECTOMY BRAS!! ALL I have to do is DRIVE TO BROOKLYN! Huh? I have one memory of EVER being in Brooklyn in my entire life. I went with two of my college friends. I believe that we went to a bar there that was previously used in a Matt Dillon movie. I learned about Brooklyn that night and I learned that if Amy ever gives up her day job, she has every bit of grit and steely-eyed determination to make it as a New York City taxi driver with just the right touch of anger for the job. It MIGHT be why she moved south. In any case, I said to the woman that I have four kids! I work! When I'm not working, I'm still attending treatment appointments. To which she said, "Ma'am? I just Googled how far Brooklyn is from you and I see that it is only 40 minutes away." You already know what my next question was. "And where are you?" The answer? "Minnesota." Well -- my reply was this, "Yes, Brooklyn is 40 minutes away from Morristown IN THEORY." So, FREE bras are over there! I've added it to my list of things to do, "Go to Brooklyn."

But in the meantime, I have finally made room in my drawer for whatever mastectomy bras I eventually acquire. I'm thinking that they are NOT going to look like the ones I donated. I was inspired by your generosity and I was able to pull out 20 bras from my drawer. And I added them to your very selfless donations, especially since there were some still with tags on them. I'm happy to announce that 206 bras are being delivered this week by ALL OF US and the company is thrilled to receive them. My sister Googled more information and she learned that homeless women often have to use belts in place of bras because they are so scarce in supply for them. And I was comforted to know that the bras will be brought to the homeless women of Newark, NJ. So the final tally was 206 bras, 3 pairs of undies, 2 pairs of socks, 1 corset, 1 slip AND 1 pony tail holder. YOU GUYS, ROCK!!!

Thank you SO very much to those that read those posts or texts of mine, took the time to clean out a drawer and drive them to my house. I don't know if I would have been able to clean out that drawer otherwise and Lord knows I've been TALKING about it for forever. I think I was trying to trick myself into it, gather the courage, realize that it's time to move on and that by TELLING you, I'd be able to get to that sad business. Thank you.

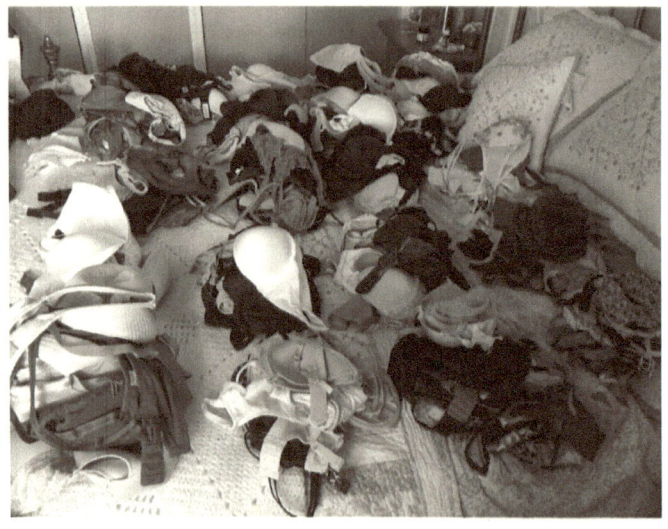

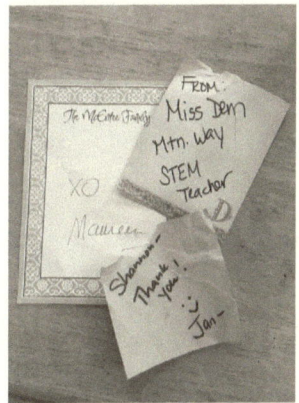

Our goal is to collect at least 500 bras by October (Breast Cancer Awareness Month). Last year, we collected 900!
Thank you!

DROP OFF OR SEND IN
NEW OR GENTLY USED BRAS
JULY THROUGH OCTOBER

We Need Your
Support!

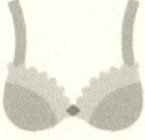

Our Goal is to Collect over 500 Bras or More
To Benefit:
The Gellman Foundation: A local organization that
will distribute them directly to homeless women in
NYC, Morristown, Dover, Newark and Jersey City.

* * * *

DENTAL STUDIES INSTITUTE
THE INSTITUTE FOR CONTINUING EDUCATION
7 Spielman Road, Fairfield, NJ 07004
(973) 808-1666

Cash/Check Donations Also Gladly Accepted
We Will Buy Bras

THE FOLLOW-UP MAMMOGRAM

January 8, 2019

YIKES!!

For the record, it doesn't get easier to go to the hospital for the first follow-up mammogram. Not at all. I've made this journey too many times. The getting out the door, getting the kids to school, the commute there, the too small parking spots, the "do they validate the parking ticket", not to mention the horrors of what's happened when you've been here before. You try to keep that on the down-low brain-wise. It's easier to worry about the waiting room TV being on too loud or when I should stop looking at the inane stuff in my phone and start that book I brought with me. I really didn't tell anyone I was coming, I can't convey the feelings I'm feeling so I'll have to keep to the details. I hate checking the box next to "Have you or anyone in your family been diagnosed with breast cancer?" The first box is "self." Check. The next ones are: Mother, sister, grandmother, aunt, etc. I am THRILLED to NOT check those boxes, but it contributes to my perplexity over this diagnosis. It's

January, but I've probably already blown the deductible. Good times. As for the other details?

The book: Little Fires Everywhere (still sitting next to me).

The waiting room TV: an ABC morning show with Ryan Seacrest (too loud).

A commercial: A Star is Born, "For Your Consideration," it says it's a "masterpiece." I still haven't seen it so I'm putting it on my list of things to get around to in 2019. Maybe it's a good idea that the TV is this loud, I'm thinking about movies to see instead of the results I will get soon. Oh, and now an item on Marie Kondo's book, the Magic of Tidying Up. And I DO have that book and the follow up book and the associated journal. I don't apologize for being a Virgo. And it's another reminder to "spark joy". Put it on the list!! But I have a public service announcement that I think should be made. You can't just buy the book and magically, your house starts tidying up. That sucks. She said it was MAGIC!!!

As for the parking ticket, it WAS validated. Good thing I'm now not worried about the four singles I left on my refrigerator that I had wanted to take with me.

The mammogram tech: I've seen her before. She just said the best thing she could've said to me right now, "That's it for the mammogram now go sit in the waiting room and then we will call you in for the ultrasound and then we will give you your results right after the ultrasound." Music to my ears. Nobody should ever have to wait for scary results.

I am also thinking about when survivorship starts. Some people say it's when they find out, so one year from finding out makes them a one year survivor. That's a valid point. For breast cancer patients, some say it's when they started chemo. Others say it's when the mastectomy removed it. I'm not sure what I think. I'm either exactly 18 months surviving or 13 months. I will keep debating this in my head, I'm sure.

All of this brain power is because I can't stop thinking about the woman that I just saw sitting in the room where I found out my news, who just had her husband called in to go into the room to meet her. I know all about what's going on in that room. But I think I need to focus on organizing my closets right now and say a prayer for her. But my thoughts drift back to the quilt that hangs on the wall in that room. That fucking quilt says that it was made in honor of a woman who fought bravely. What the fuck is that? THAT is where they put someone to tell them news that changes their life instantly? That someone before her didn't make it, someone who may have sat in that very same room? The absurdity amazes me. At the very least, move the quilt somewhere else. Or how about this? Whomever quilted in somebody's honor should have given it to someone that actually needs a quilt.

At least I did see something inspirational. In the elevator, someone has stenciled. "Inhale courage. Exhale fear." Okay, I'm following directions. Inhale, exhale. Inhale, exhale.

Here's what I have going in my favor. When I had the mammogram after chemo and before the mastectomy, everything looked good and there were just residual leftovers to deal with in surgery. Chemo had done a "tremendous" job. But it has always stayed in my head that it wasn't 100 percent clear.

And now the same ultrasound tech just came to get me, the one that dealt the news last year. She's very nice. She said I looked familiar. I don't know if I'll remind her that I was the one sitting here sobbing a year and a half ago. Never mind; I did just thank her. And she asked how I was doing. I gave her the update. And I told her it doesn't get easier to come here. And she said it's not going to. But she did say this, and I will take this with me, "This is the first time. You've probably been thinking about it for at least a couple of days. Each time you will still think about it but maybe it'll be less days each time." She had gone through something similar, she conveyed. And while it never leaves her mind, she said she really only worries about it the day before now.

I also just saw the same Nurse Navigator; she gave me a friendly hello. She had held me up while my world fell apart. "Hi, Nurse Navigator, I remember you and I thank you for what you've done for me." She ran by before I could say anything, but I repeated it in my head. Hopefully she felt the blessings I wished for her.

I have five red jasper crystals in the front pocket of my jeans right now, I only had to disrobe from the waist up. I read that they're lucky for Virgos. I even soaked them in salt water for 24 hours to clean them and had them "charge" by the light of the sun and the full moon. Sounds crazy, right? Well. I. Am. Crazy. I dare you not to be crazy after a year and a half like this. I triple dog dare you. I'm at the point where if someone told me that standing on my head and spitting wooden nickels would help, I'd start amassing them and get out my yoga mat.

Journaling has been saving my life. I'm still up and at it every morning, three pages. Yesterday was the first day in months that I missed. It was Zach's birthday. And the birthday boy requested my pumpkin pancakes for breakfast. And I had an early morning oncologist appointment. I carried that thing around with me all day, I was really planning to get to it but I was already too tired to write by the time I got settled for the night. There was no way I was missing it today. It clears the junk out of my head in the wee hours of the morning.

As for the year long medicine I'm on, it's still kicking my butt. Literally and figuratively. I often have a toddler bedtime. As weird as it sounds, a cholesterol lowering medication has been found to positively affect the side effects. I took it for one month despite having great cholesterol and it really did the trick. It has been a game changer but not for the fatigue. The fatigue is relentless. My kids tuck me in lately, not the other way around. I may look normal tonight. You may see me. But if I'm up, it comes from somewhere, so you might not see me for several days. I often feel almost normal, but it is squeezed down into a much more condensed window. I follow a private Facebook group of women on this crazy medicine -- almost all say that they feel totally normal again about three days after they stop. Today is day 131. And, yes, I know which day it is every single day. I ask Siri to divide the day by 389. Today I am 33.67 percent done. Since I started at a low dose and ramped up to full dose over several weeks, and missed taking it once or twice, that's the amount of days I need to serve.

So, by now I've been laying here waiting for quite a while, post mammography, pre ultrasound. Why, you ask? I'm always interested in the curiosities of modern medicine. They are looking for something. A second prescription. It was decided upon late last night to add this second prescription and it almost didn't happen. I was told that my appointment would be for a mammogram and ultrasound of my right breast. OK, great. But what about an ultrasound of the left? "No, we don't usually do that. You had a simple mastectomy all should be fine." But the cancer was on my left. "Nope. It should be fine then. We will just be doing the right." and a "It's always done this way." Nope. Nope. Nope.

In all fairness, if a woman has a single mastectomy because that's where cancer was found, how in the world does she leave happy to find out that it's STILL not in the other breast but without anyone looking at the side that caused alarm? The panic? The nightmare? I need to know. One missed cell could change the course of events. I don't want to wait until I have symptoms. And so they are looking for the prescription that was faxed over late last night. This makes total sense to me. I don't know why it doesn't to them. But, wait -- the ultrasound tech just said to me, "Some women do it the way you're doing. This is the way I'd do it, too. But, you didn't hear that from me." Nope. I didn't hear it from you. I heard it from me. Again, the curiosities of modern medicine.

"Everything looks good. That's great. You're free to go." Oh, thank you, God. Thank you, thank you, thank you, God. Now I just have to find my newly validated parking ticket and I'm out of here. But, first, I text Tom, my mom, my sister and my aunt. "Mammogram and ultrasound of right: clear. Ultrasound of left: clear. I can't find the right emoji to attach, but the feeling is similar to letting out a toxic breath you've been holding too long." They need an, "Oh, thank God" emoji. The prayer hands are there but I need a face that would express that deep emotion.

You might have just heard me peeling out. I'm OUTTA here!

Oh, and Claire got me a new phone case. 😊 :) A greater truth would be unknown to me. 2016 changed me. 2017 broke me. 2018 opened my eyes. 2019 I'm coming back.

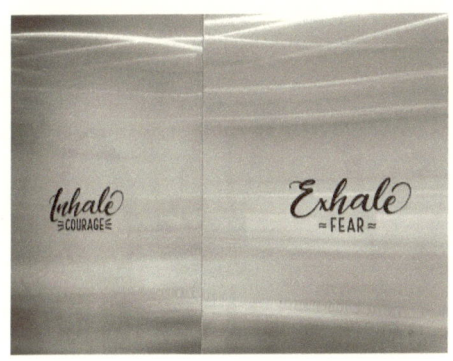

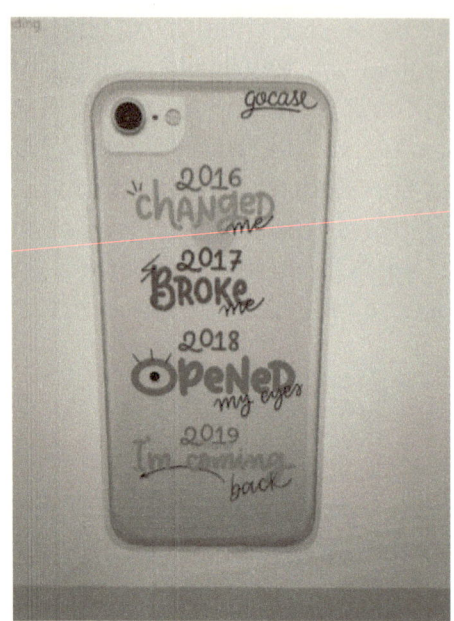

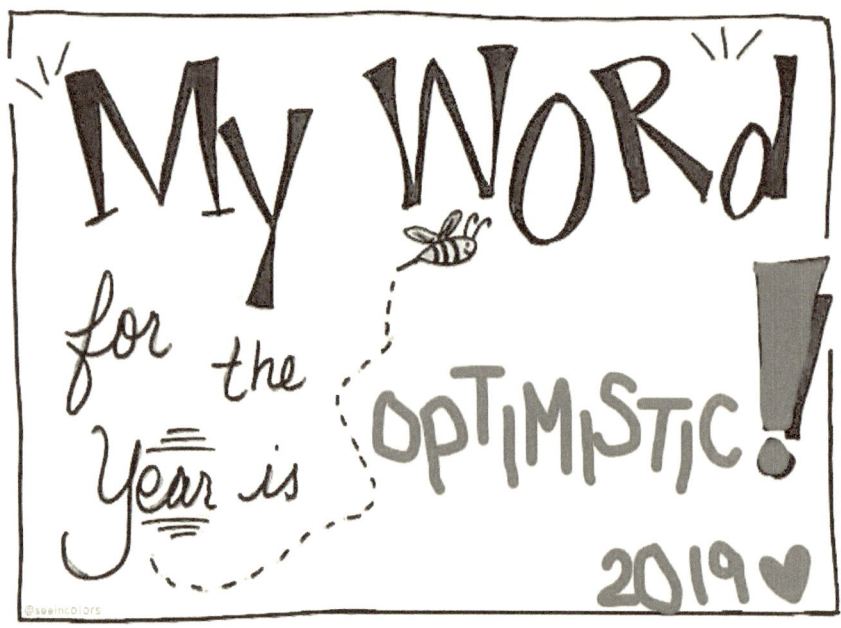

SIGNS

APRIL 1, 2019

Sign, sign, everywhere a sign, blocking out the scenery, breakin' my mind

Do this, don't do that, can't you read the sign...

C hildren of the 80's would say that "Signs" is sung by Tesla. Children of the 70's would say that it's Five Man Electrical Band.

I'm emotional today. I didn't really start out that way. It even takes me by surprise. Is it the spring look to the sky? It's definitely not the feel (Brrr. What an April Fool's joke, a wind chill of 22 in the northeast today). Is it the angst of continued treatment? The article I saw this morning that said, "Most cancer comes back because the person's body adapts to the medication." Is it because I'm sooooo tired of the fatigue that comes over me like a wave? The hot flashes? The way I know the nuances of my bathrooms now better than I did before?

I began my seventh bottle of twelve of the dreaded medicine I started in September. I am halfway done, still gunning for that September 21st end date. I know that many women don't finish it due to the quality of life issues it brings. In a private Facebook group I'm in for it, a woman recently asked, "Does anyone ever skip a day because they are so tired of the way it makes them feel?" People answered, "Oh, yes. I stopped it for a vacation. I stopped it because I couldn't take the side effects, yadda, yadda, yadda." My answer was simple, "I have forgotten to take it a couple of times, but it makes me sick to have to add it to the end date."

Symptoms continue to be, besides the fatigue and bathroom trips, fingernail infections, paper thin nails, UTIs. A patient told me the other day that she "couldn't wait until menopause." My experience is that I hate the flatline feeling, the loss of libido, the hot flashes. I'd take a menstrual cycle any day, if only for that beautiful mid-cycle feeling. The ups that balance the downs. Menopause is similar to purgatory in my opinion. It's the kind of a thing that is always coming for the ladies, all the ladies, but no one wants to be forced into it.

Another feeling of purgatory came up at my yearly follow-up with my surgeon recently. I asked her about what I was dealing with (you will never see me put the words "MY" and "cancer" together again). I had hormone positive breast cancer, which has great treatment options but has a risk of recurring later in life, approximately 30 percent of the time. But I also had that inflammatory component of the breast cancer. The risk of inflammatory breast cancer returning comes earlier, 64 percent of the time, within five years. Does it feel a little "damned if you do, damned if you don't?" YUP.

I had a conversation with someone close to me once. Her husband had been diagnosed with a couple of things that made him stop drinking, stop smoking and start eating a more healthy diet. He died two years later. She said to me, "You know what? When I think of how miserable he was in those last two years? I think he should have eaten the fucking hotdogs." So, there's THAT to consider. Personally, I think of lips and assholes when I think of hotdogs but I think you catch my drift.

Weirdly enough, a small dose of antidepressants actually combatted the hot flashes and brought me up a little, back to where I feel comfortable staying "on the sunny side, always on the sunny side" a song that the girls from my Girl Scout troop learned at camp last year. So this IS NOT a dismal post. Think of it as an observational post. No judgements needed, just what the hell is exactly going on, "the latest from here," if you will.

Whenever I write one of these posts, I finish it and I think, "DONE NOW! I have NOTHING left to say. There!" And, then I find myself percolating thoughts, concepts, that I need to address, get out of me and I think of the famous line from Hamilton: "How do you write like you need it to survive. NONSTOP."

So what happens in the year after the one year diagnosis survival for a cancer patient? Well, they may have felt better the day before their diagnosis than they do now. Side effects abound; their retirement fund may be empty; their kids might need extra special care.

These kids have been scared for a long time. They need space; they need to work things out; they may be acting out. These are typical kid things but exacerbated by a REALLY BIG SCARY THING. An observation is that they are not bringing you everything that's bothering them. They are afraid of adding to your worries, given the circumstances, not that they should be. The patient might be TOTALLY CRAZED with getting things off a list of experiences that they want for their kids: the first concert, the first major league baseball game, the first this, the first that, none of it indulgent when compared to the rest of the northeasterners' kids. SICK TO DEATH that you are encouraging your kids to take SATS, etc., and the uber-rich are paying their kids ways in. Thankful that FAFSAs will take into account the year without a salary, but, still scared of not having enough money to pay for college.

The cancer patient might be mourning their lost libido. They are in mourning for life as they remember it. Another summer coming, another mastectomy bathing suit. Those are the bad days, but there are more good days than bad now. The surgeon was amazed at my post-radiation skin at my yearly follow-up; said it didn't look like it had been irradiated (thank you aloe and coconut oil).

When people ask my secret -- it's no secret -- journaling, meditating, juicing. I like to "JUICE THE RAINBOW" -- red apples, orange carrots, yellow lemons, green ANYTHING, purple beets, with some brown ginger. I mix it with Berry Kombucha, for the best tasting vegetable soda you've ever had. It's sort of a joke; it's sort of not a joke. I have only gotten one kid to try it, Zach, post swim meet and dehydrated to the max. He said, "This is so bad and so good at the same time."

We adopted a dog for all the right reasons you should have for getting a dog. But the best part has been giving us something else to talk about. In weird NJ news, Dixie is NOT a lab, like we thought we brought home, but a Plott Hound, complete with that hound sense of drive. I fantasize about letting her loose at the deer sometimes but Plott Hounds are hunt driven and it "often ends tragically" if they get off leash. They will follow a scent for miles and not stop to look both ways. No off leash for us.

There are LOTS AND LOTS of things swirling in my head today, but I was good this morning.

And then emotions started in the car, on my way to work this morning. I was SUPER PSYCHED to tune into a radio station playing Ariana Grande's No Tears Left to Cry.

Right now, I'm in a state of mind

I wanna be in like all the time

Ain't got no tears left to cry

So I'm pickin' it up, pickin' it up

I'm lovin', I'm livin', I'm pickin' it up

Lovin', I'm livin', so we turnin' up

Yeah, we turnin' it up

My kids have come to hate when that song comes on in the car. I sing it so much louder than they want AND I like to throw in some demonstrative moves. It is SO fun that when their complaints hit a dull roar, it's almost the exact time when I can sing,

"CAN'T STOP, SO SHUT YOUR MOUTH" It gives such GREAT pleasure EVERY TIME that I'm smiling to myself right now.

So I was good! The sun was shining. And then Rachel Platten's Fight Song came on. I was STILL good.

This is my fight song

Take back my life song

Prove I'm alright song

My power's turned on

Starting right now I'll be strong

I'll play my fight song

And I don't really care if nobody else believes

'Cause I've still got a lot of fight left in me

and then.

AND THEN:

"It's been two years, I miss my home"

And it made me burst out crying. Instantly! Damn hormones. Or lack of damn hormones. This week is 1-3/4 years since our lives changed. Close enough to two years and it's good...and scary...and emotional...and I think of all of the gifts that have been given to me since then, and what I've learned and what I need to pass on to my kids as wisdom. And the things I still want to, need to, take care of for my family, and I start to spin a little bit.

So I try to think of what I need to do today. I'm looking for a pink

Rubbermaid or Sterilite container, the big one...and I'm heading home and throwing LOTS of stuff in it...a wig, a styrofoam head (there are things that you just don't want to have to buy again, IF...and let's just leave it at that). I think it's time to pass along the talisman that one of my BFFs gave me when I started this fight. The cancer beanies will get donated. I never wore them anyway. Don't get too close to me this afternoon. It's going to be a frenzy and I don't want to throw any innocent bystanders in by mistake.

And that's ALL what I was thinking on Route 24 this morning, listening to Fight Song, crying, but wearing my new sunglasses. I was thinking that I have a plan for today and it's going to be okay. And then, up ahead, I see a tractor trailer with gigantic letters spelling out THE END up ahead. This was a sign and for some reason, I feel the need to PASS this FUCKING TRUCK. You see? I can't chase this truck all day. It can't get off an exit before me. It can't stay ahead of me. Don't worry, I was still getting passed by careless drivers, texting. But as I was finally gaining on this tractor trailer, there was now a dump truck next to me, and THAT one says, "Jesus is my guide" on the back. Another sign.

It's April first. I keep hearing that April is called "Angel Month." I don't know why yet. And my daffodils are coming up. And Mercury is out of retrograde. And, I passed the truck that says "The End" this morning. I NEEDED to. I was POSSESSED until I did. And, as I did, Coldplay's Clocks came on:

> You are, you are
>
> Confusion that never stops
>
> The closing walls and the ticking clocks gonna
>
> Come back and take you home
>
> I could not stop, that you now know, singing
>
> Come out upon my seas
>
> Cursed missed opportunities am I
>
> A part of the cure

Or am I part of the disease, singing...

You are...you are...

And I decide to be part of the cure. And I decide that for future commutes, I will go back to my classic rock stations, intermixed with a healthy dose of AM newsradio that I spend an abnormal amount of time waiting for "traffic and weather together" and then forgetting to listen to while it's on. Anything but this, "highs are too high and lows are too low" music station. At least for now.

This afternoon I will pack up that pink Sterilite box with breast cancer paraphernalia that, in truth, I never want to see again and in a THICK, BLACK Sharpie, I'm going to write, "Do not open. There is but no need. - The Management." It's going to go on a shelf in the basement pushed ALL the way to the back. And then I'm going to go drink the best vegetable soda you ever drank in your life. And I will walk my Plott Hound. And call to make an appointment for a haircut. It's been one year since my last haircut exactly, this month. AND THEN, I will pick up the kids from school. And THEN, my darlings, "How was your day? I missed you while you were at school today."

Addendum: A 16-gallon pink Sterilite container was found at Watchung Walmart at 1:42 p.m. today, April 1, 2019. It cost $5.78 and I'm considering it money well spent. The End.

Dr. Shannon M. Mulvey

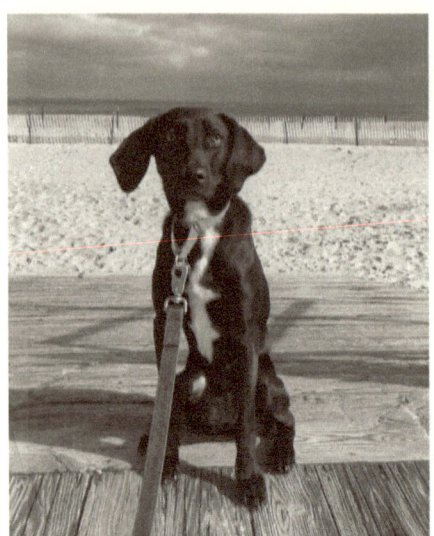
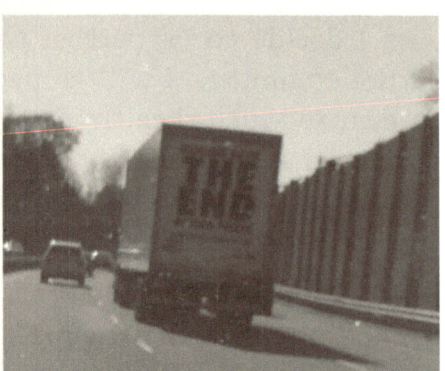

LOVE LIVES HERE

July 7, 2017? No, July 7, 2019.

Just an ordinary day...

I t's a day of good news for me!! I ALMOST MISSED it but I'm both glad I almost missed it and equally glad I didn't...

Here's the AWESOME news -- I am a two year survivor today. It humbles me. It scares me. It motivates me. It inspires me. I continue to waver between celebrating survivability on the day I was diagnosed versus the day it was sent packing via surgery, 5 months later. I will celebrate both.

Here's the even better news. I got up early today. I journaled my requisite 3 pages. I gave thanks. I considered the most important things I had to take care of today. I started laundry. I filled out medical paperwork for my kids. I started making bacon for breakfast for my older guys who are returning to staff camp for the week today. I tried to wake one of them up; I will try again in a bit. I started making green smoothies for the week -- assembling them in mason jars to just add liquid to and then blend in the mornings. I petted Dixie for a few minutes. I did some other more boring things not worth mentioning. And then I wrote the date on something. 7/7/17, I wrote out. As I said two years ago, I liked the alliteration of that date. At the time. It's weird that the surgery was on 12/12/17. But today, I realized that -- WAIT -- it is 2019!! Why did I just write 2017???? Oh, yeah...to be reminded from the universe, my subconscious, the powers that be that today is just a normal summer morning. It was the most abnormal day of my life on a Friday, two years ago. It is obviously a Sunday this year and I give thanks. I have three more months of this oral chemotherapy. I DO have normal days, like today. But I have abnormal days, too. I slept until 10:30 am yesterday, not out of luxuriousness. I had to stay somewhat close to home yesterday. I felt nauseated and out of sync. I am inspired by a blog post from Rachel Hollis. #LAST90DAYS. She reserves this concept for the October, November and December season in which she kicks into gear WAY before deciding to change her life on January 1. But, I'm adopting it for the last 90 days of this awful medicine. Hence the green smoothie factory assembly line. 90 days brings me to September 30 and October 1. Which, interestingly, is Rosh Hashanah. Year 5780, to be exact. I'm not Jewish but I love the idea of ending this medicine on a "new year", as it will be one for me as well. St. Patrick's Day celebrating is obviously a must here. But, after all, our family always celebrates Chinese New Year, too, and we're not Chinese. So, Happy Year of the Earth Pig, Year 4716, while I'm celebrating. I will be throwing in ALL of the celebrations I can think of!! You know what? Sometimes I make grandiose assumptions like about not being Jewish or Chinese. Only I know my ethnic background. We don't know Tom's and therefore, his half of the kids' ethnic backgrounds so I won't assume. We will continue to celebrate everything!!

The days have been busy. Thrown into the normal mumbo-jumbo have been some symptoms. They were scary. They made me not feel good. It became an appointment with a specialist which became an ultrasound appointment which became a biopsy appointment which became wait for a week and pretend that you are only worried about getting your kid to swim practice on time. Nod your head in polite solidarity when someone says to you that the end of the school year is so stressful. "Yes," I say. "It is so stressful."

And then the news came on a Friday morning instead of having to wait through the weekend. All clear. I still don't feel terrific -- but I'm hanging my hat on that it's the medication and it's many known and common side effects and that there are 90 last days of them. Thank you, God. So I will keep casually seizing the day over here in case I can't tomorrow. I will keep making plans, because today I have no reason to think I won't see them through. I will keep cranking the Foo Fighters.

And another best was another day with the beautiful ladies of Beautiful Self dedicated to getting breast cancer survivors back on their feet. One of the most fun days of my life. When they heard what was going on in my life, they said, "You know what? If you have all of that going on, you don't have to do this for us." I said, "ARE YOU KIDDING???? THAT'S WHY I HAVE TO DO IT!!" I will gratefully consider ANY and ALL breaks from reality right now. Except crack. And I got a fantastic necklace from A. Jaffe out of the deal. It was like icing on the cake because I didn't need anything to make that day more fun than it was. The necklace shows a map of our neighborhood, with a diamond placed at our address where I live with my family, where love lives. Which is why I had inscribed on the back -- "Love Lives Here. S, T, S, Z, C & M". Chaos also lives here. Glorious chaos reigns supreme in a good way. But that didn't fit on the necklace.

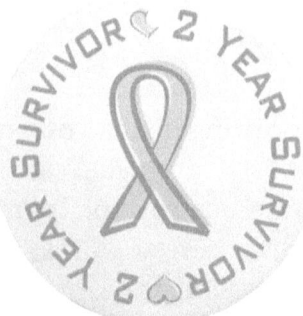

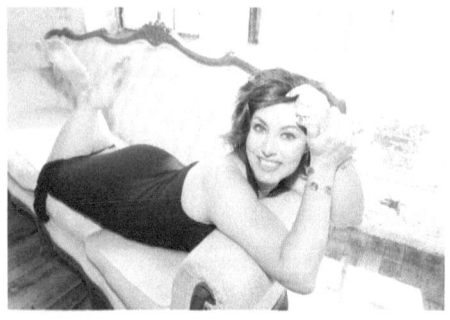

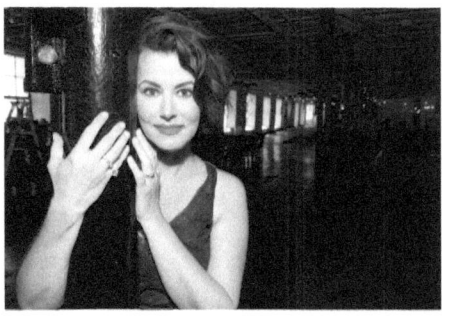

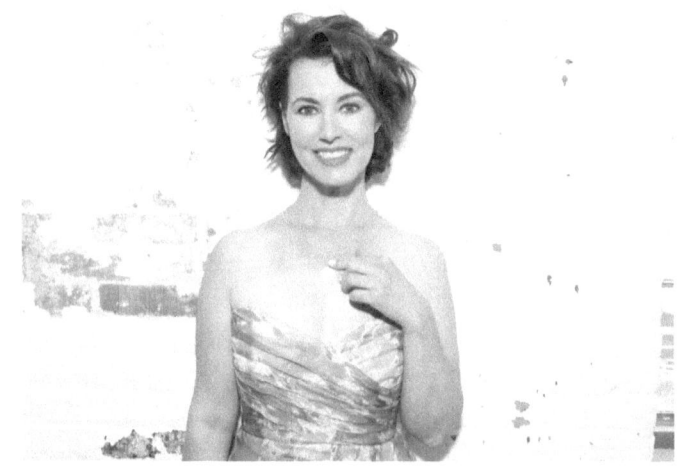

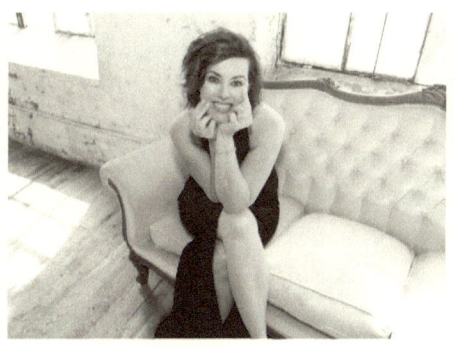

THE END.

April 1...no year...

YEAH, RIGHT!

The End???! I'm just kidding. Happy April Fool's Day! There is no end to cancer survival. I get fooled EVERY SINGLE DAY. Like the movie Groundhog Day. There's only a beginning to cancer, a continuum from there and I'm just getting started. I even plan to keep adding chapters to this public diary. I still have three more months of this SHITTY medication and sometimes my doctors talk about taking my estrogen producing ovaries. Reconstruction possibly someday. A year ago, I would have said I would DEFINITELY reconstruct and I probably still will. But there are days when I think -- if I have to wait THIS long for reconstruction, will I get used to it and desire NOT to put my body through another recovery process? An implant is not in the picture for me due to the inflammatory component of this beast. That means they would only be taking my own stuffing out of one place and putting it in another place. The recovery time is substantial. I am told this may be OUT OF POCKET as it is possibly ELECTIVE. CAN YOU BELIEVE THAT RIDICULOUSNESS?? Note to self: start fighting insurance companies soon. After all, I've done it before. After I had my FOURTH CHILD, the insurance company that we had FOR YEARS wouldn't pay for the labor and delivery. As usual, many hours of sitting on the phone later, it was discovered that I was in their system listed as a MAN. Now DESPITE what people may say about me, I am not a man. That thought makes me laugh out loud. This company covered three prior pregnancies. And someone rubberstamped it UNPAID instead of looking for the story of my male pregnancy on the cover of TIME magazine. Or calling the provider. AND THEN, there was the time that my appendectomy was not covered because it was considered elective surgery. Yeah, it was. I elected to live that day. Okay storm Washington, D.C. just got added to the list. It is not always easy to find clothes right now, even if I was not a very revealing dresser in the first place. Dresses, v-necks and tank tops don't always look right, because they don't fall right. And there's really no such thing as a sexy prosthetic bra. Looking for one harks back to the time that I tried to find pretty nursing bras. Taking my stuffing from another place adds to the number of areas that would need to heal. I cringe at the thought of people congratulating me on getting "a boob job". And could I really be an adept chiropractor missing muscles from my traps or my abdomen? Missing my left chest muscle is a notable loss when it comes to treating patients. We shall see. It's all part of the journey. A road that I didn't want to take but I am trying to learn new things along the way. I didn't have a choice.

As usual, thank you my loves for lending an ear. I hope it helps in any sort of way, whether you are a survivor, a thriver, a caregiver or just a rocker. Or you are on a journey that you did not choose. I know getting it out of my head helped me. And if it doesn't help you, just consider these the ravings of a lunatic and...rock on.

> *Carry on, my wayward son,*
>
> *For there'll be peace when you are done*
>
> *Lay your weary head to rest*
>
> *Don't you cry no more.*
>
>   - Kansas

Oh, and peace out and word to the mutha...

Love always,

Dr. Shannon M. Mulvey

Shannon

XOXOX

———————————

MY BEAST MODE PLAYLIST, IN NO
PARTICULAR ORDER.

Beautiful....Christina Aguilera
Best of You...Foo Fighters
Fighter...Christina Aguilera
Can't Hold Us...Macklemore & Ryan Lewis
I Gotta Feeling...The Black Eyed Peas
It's Not My Time...3 Doors Down
Lose Yourself...Eminem
Unwritten...Natasha Bedingfield
You Gotta Be...Des'ree
Survivor...Destiny's Child
I Won't Back Down...Tom Petty
Life is Beautiful...Sixx: A.M.
Safe and Sound...Sheryl Crow
All My Life...Foo Fighters
Everlong...Foo Fighters
Learn to Fly...Foo Fighters
Times Like These...Foo Fighters
Dreams...Van Halen
Praying...Kesha
Walk...Foo Fighters
Good Feeling...Flo Rida
No Tears Left to Cry...Ariana Grande
Fight Song...Rachel Platten
Bust a Move...Young MC
Dreams...Van Halen
FEMALE...Sampa the Great
All I Do is Win...DJ Khaled
It's Not My Time...3 Doors Down
ALL Foo Fighters, ALL Taylor Swift, All Black Keys and ALLHamilton, The Musical.

Thank yous and Acknowledgements....

The list of people to thank is endless, there is nowhere to start and there is nowhere to end. It goes without saying that my husband Tom, my children, Sam, Zach, Claire and Max, my parents, Nadine and Tom Mulvey, my siblings, Melissa and Mike Imparato, Todd and Paige Mulvey, my Aunt Valerie and Uncle Ron Dryka, my Grandmother Joan Mabie and my mother-in-law MaryAnn Boverini were the ones who caught me when I fell. They fell, too, but still somehow managed to hold me up.

My place of employment, Gordon Family Injury Center, for never putting any pressure on me to come back to work, even though I was gone for a year. And the ladies there, all the ladies. Men, too.

The Pittaro Family, Susan, Justin, JT and Allie, who formed my team. Family.

The Foo Fighters, obvs.

My surgeon, Dr. Leah Gendler, my oncologist, Dr. Jason Levitz, my Radiation Oncologist, Dr. Mona Karim and all of their caring staffs. I absolutely have no idea how they do this every day.

Breast Imaging Nurse Navigator Renee Trambert, Oncology Social Worker Kristy Case, Integrative Oncology Coordinator Jean Marie Rosone. All ready with tissues and words of wisdom for the newly diagnosed.

Marla Jan...Author Diana Lopez,for having an age appropriate book, *Ask My Mood Ring How I Feel*, talking about mastectomies that showed up in my daughter's hands at just the right time.

Author Sarah Young and her book *Jesus Calling*. Facebook savage Shelly Melton, who has more bravery than anyone I could ever imagine. The volunteers of Knitted Knockers and especially Jean Scully who knitted two knockers for me, made to order...Cancer Warrioress blogger, Tara Coyote and especially her "Healing Heartbreak", which spoke to me...Tiny Buddha and their Facebook wisdom, Jenn Brenner, poettess. Caitlin Feeley of the Dread Pirate Khan blog and her "The Mountain Lion" work of art. The Diva for a Day organization, Beth at Morris Plains Maid Pro.

Special thanks to Judy Mennonna, who took me under her wing and linked me up with the incredible volunteers of Minnette's Angels charity, especially Suzy Grosso, for breast cancer patients and also to Beautiful Self and their breast cancer charity -- the amazing Jillian Rezo and Michele Bonacorte, all whom I will love forever. As I always say about Judy -- she loves fiercely and she was the first breast cancer survivor that took me in to mentor.

Also thanks to April Heather, Taylor Swift and her free tickets for area Girl Scouts, any Inflammatory Breast Cancer warriors, forever explaining that this is not your average breast cancer. Not that ANY are average, IBC just REALLY isn't. The Gellman Foundation and Institute of Continuing Education in Fairfield, NJ, making me aware of just how many homeless women must go braless. And, thanks to Rachel Hollis and her intrepid bravery, making it her business to lift up women and thanks to A. Jaffe for my beautiful Maps necklace.

To my editor, Nancy Verga and to my graphic designer, who shall remain nameless for now.

Lastly, my friends who showed up with tissues and books and trinkets and giftcards and bravery, in no particular order Lisa Foley, BethAnne Steneck, Stephanie Halcomb, Amy Loria, Leigh Smith, Lori Bergeron, Kristen Coughlin, Rachel Sambrowski, Angela Lewis, Tracy Dragos, Diana Fonseca, Amie Hyman, Janit London, Paula Lalin, Karla Lortie, Karen Riley -- all of these ladies had their hands holding the net for me...Thank you all for blessing me. I would remiss if I didn't mention the Community of Morris Plains. I can't imagine having had to navigate this mess anywhere but here, the Community of Caring.

I just know I'm missing people from this list and for that I'm sorry. Every single kindness blessed me and my family.

www.ingramcontent.com/pod-product-compliance
Lightning Source LLC
Chambersburg PA
CBHW020317290526
45785CB00007B/2829